try it!

15-MINUTE
FITNESS

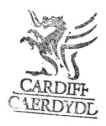

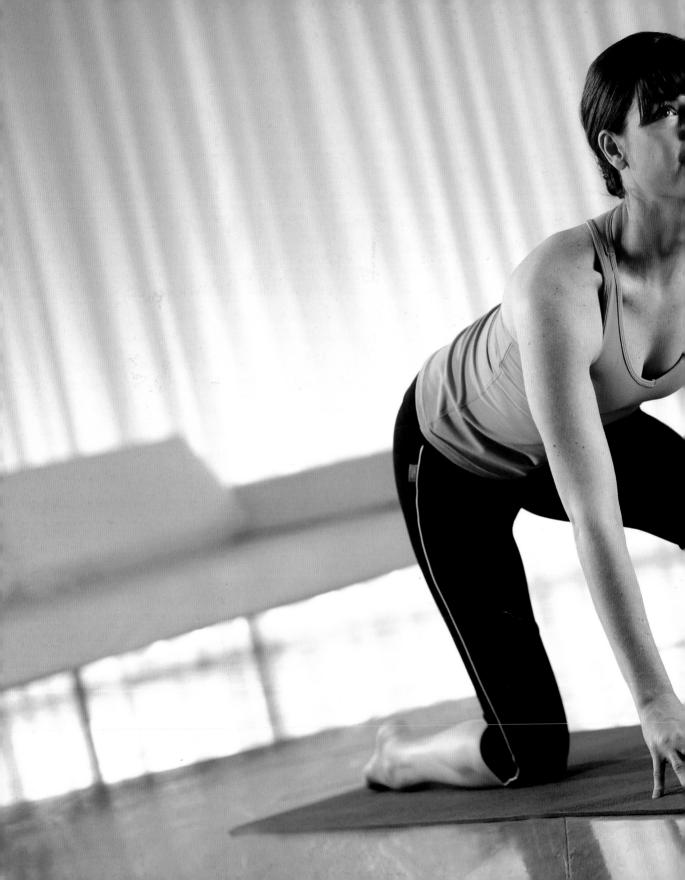

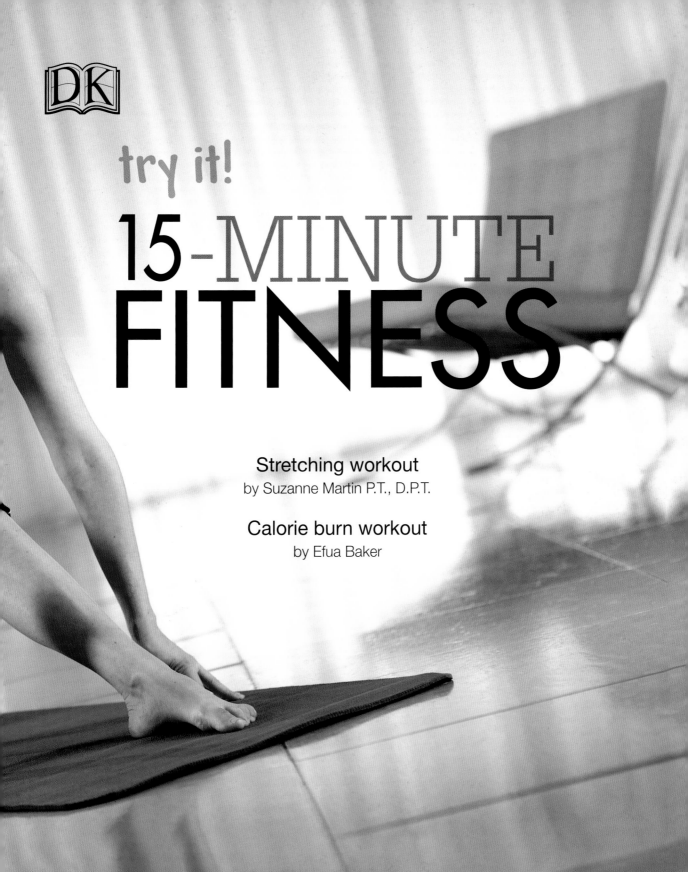

DK

try it!

15-MINUTE
FITNESS

Stretching workout
by Suzanne Martin P.T., D.P.T.

Calorie burn workout
by Efua Baker

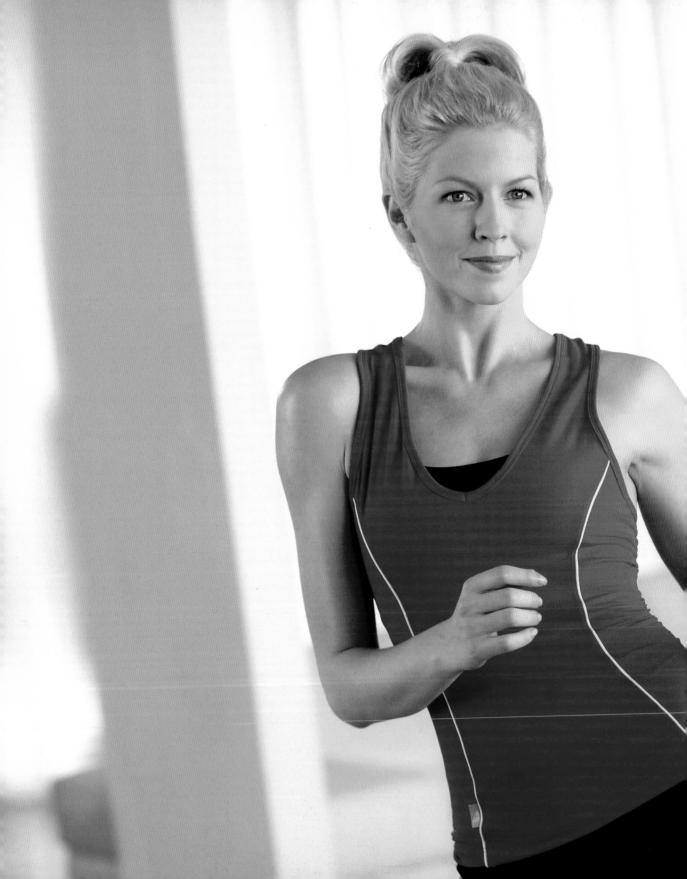

contents

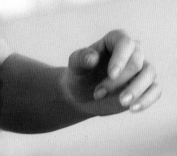

>> how to use this book

The programmes in this book have each been specially designed to give you a well-rounded workout in 15 minutes. With step-by-step photographs and clear instructions for each exercise, these routines are the closest you can get to having a personal trainer right by your side.

In each of the 15-minute programmes, the photographs capture the essence of the exercises in simple step-by-step images. Some exercises require two or three images, while others only need one. Certain exercises contain smaller inset photos that depict the first step, or starting position. This is to make the sequence clearer for you to follow. You will also find targeted

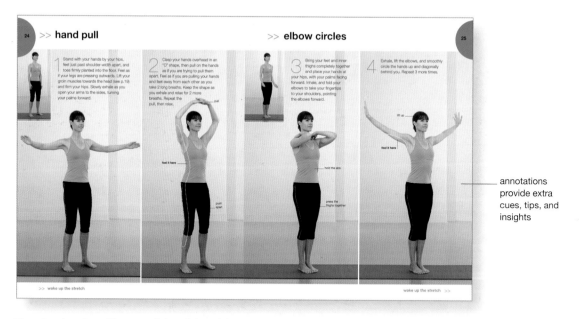

annotations provide extra cues, tips, and insights

The step-by-steps These work from left to right as you follow the step-by-step exercises. Be certain you understand the beginning and end positions before progressing.

"feel-it-here" graphics (marked by white dotted lines) on specific exercises. These are intended to emphasize the fact that there is always a different area of the body to focus on.

The at-a-glance charts

The at-a-glance charts help you see each programme in full view. Once you've practised each move thoroughly, these charts will become invaluable. Use them as a quick reference to trim your practice down to a succinct 15 minutes.

Exercising effectively

The programmes in Stretching workout are suitable to practise every day if you wish to do so. The programmes in Calorie burn workout should be performed with a rest day in between. Muscles need one full day of rest in between strength-training workouts, as the recovery time is just as important to the development of muscle as the exertion. For maximum results, you can do 30 minutes of moderate cardio exercise, such as swimming, walking, or cycling, on your "off" days.

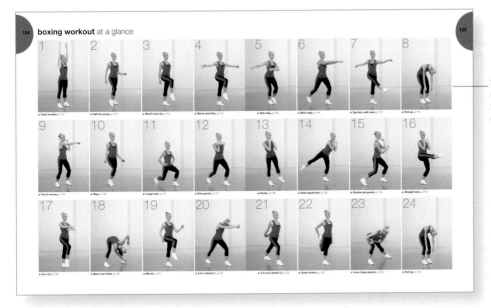

the at-a-glance charts show all the main steps of the programme

At-a-glance charts These will help guide you along once you no longer need the step-by-step images. It is best to review the full programme before beginning.

>> **safety** issues

Before you start any training programme, you must make sure that it is safe for you to begin. First, take the PAR-Q questionnaire on the opposite page to see if you should check with your doctor before beginning. Remember, it's always wise to consult your doctor if you're suffering from an illness or any injuries.

Test your fitness

When starting a fitness programme, it's useful to see how your muscular fitness measures up by counting how many repetitions you can perform or how many seconds you can hold a contraction. The three exercises shown here will assess your muscular endurance in the lower, middle, and upper body. Record your results, noting the date, and after three months of training, repeat the tests. When you reassess yourself, perform the same version of the exercise. Before attempting the exercises, warm up first by moving briskly for five minutes.

If you are just beginning to exercise, or coming back to it after a long break, you may prefer to perform your first assessment after two or three months of exercising on a regular basis.

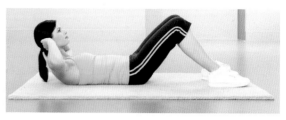

Middle body *Crunch with Scoop*
Count how many crunches you can do consecutively without resting. This is not a full sit-up. Lift your head and shoulders no higher than 30 degrees off the mat.

Your score

Excellent	50 reps or more
Good	35–49 reps
Fair	20–34 reps
Poor	20 reps or less

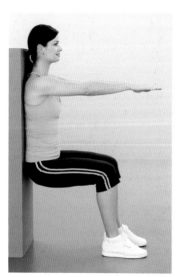

Lower body

Wall Squat
Slide down until your thighs are parallel to the floor and hold the position for as long as you can. (If you cannot slide all the way down, go as far as you can.)

Your score

Excellent	90 seconds or more
Good	60 seconds
Fair	30 seconds
Poor	less than 30 seconds

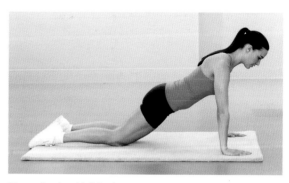

Upper body *Half Push-up*
Inhale as you bend your elbows, lowering your chest to the floor. Exhale as you push up to the starting position. Count how many you can do consecutively without a rest.

Your score

Excellent	20 reps or more
Good	15–19 reps
Fair	10–14 reps
Poor	10 reps or less

PAR-Q AND YOU A questionnaire for people aged 15 to 69 Physical Activity Readiness Questionnaire – PAR-Q (revised 2002)

Regular physical activity is fun and healthy, and increasingly more people are starting to become more active every day. Being more active is perfectly safe for most people. However, some people should check with their doctor before they start becoming much more physically active than they are already.

If you are planning to become much more physically active than you are now, start by answering the seven questions in the box below. If you are between the ages of 15 and 69, the PAR-Q will tell you if you should check with your doctor before you start. If you are over 69 years of age, and you are not used to being very active, check with your doctor.

Common sense is your best guide when you answer these questions. Please read the questions carefully and answer each one honestly: check YES or NO.

YES	NO	
☐	☐	**1** Has your doctor ever said that you have a heart condition <u>and</u> that you should only do physical activity recommended by a doctor?
☐	☐	**2** Do you feel pain in your chest when you do physical activity?
☐	☐	**3** In the past month, have you had chest pain when you were not doing physical activity?
☐	☐	**4** Do you lose your balance because of dizziness or do you ever lose consciousness?

YES	NO	
☐	☐	**5** Do you have a bone or joint problem (for example, back, knee, or hip) that could possibly be made worse by a marked change in your physical activity?
☐	☐	**6** Is your doctor currently prescribing drugs (for example, water pills) for your blood pressure or heart condition?
☐	☐	**7** Do you know of any other reason why you should not do physical activity?

If you answered YES to one or more questions

Talk with your doctor by phone or in person BEFORE you start becoming much more physically active or BEFORE you have a fitness appraisal.
Tell your doctor about the PAR-Q and which questions you answered YES.
• You may be able to do any activity you want – as long as you start slowly and build up gradually. Or, you may need to restrict your activities to those which are safe for you. Talk with your doctor about the kinds of activities you wish to participate in and follow his/her advice.
• Find out which community programmes are going to prove safe and helpful for you.

If you answered NO to all questions

If you answered NO honestly to all PAR-Q questions, you can be reasonably sure that you can:
• start becoming much more physically active – begin slowly and build up gradually. This is the safest and easiest way to go.
• take part in a fitness appraisal – this is an excellent way to determine your basic fitness so that you can plan the best way for you to live actively. It is also highly recommended that you have your blood pressure evaluated. If your reading is over 144/94, talk with your doctor before you start becoming much more physically active.

DELAY BECOMING MUCH MORE ACTIVE:
• if you are not feeling well because of a temporary illness such as a cold or a fever – wait until you feel better
• if you are or may be pregnant – talk to your doctor before you start becoming more active.

PLEASE NOTE:
If your health changes so that you then answer YES to any of the above questions, tell your fitness or health professional. Ask whether you should change your physical activity plan.

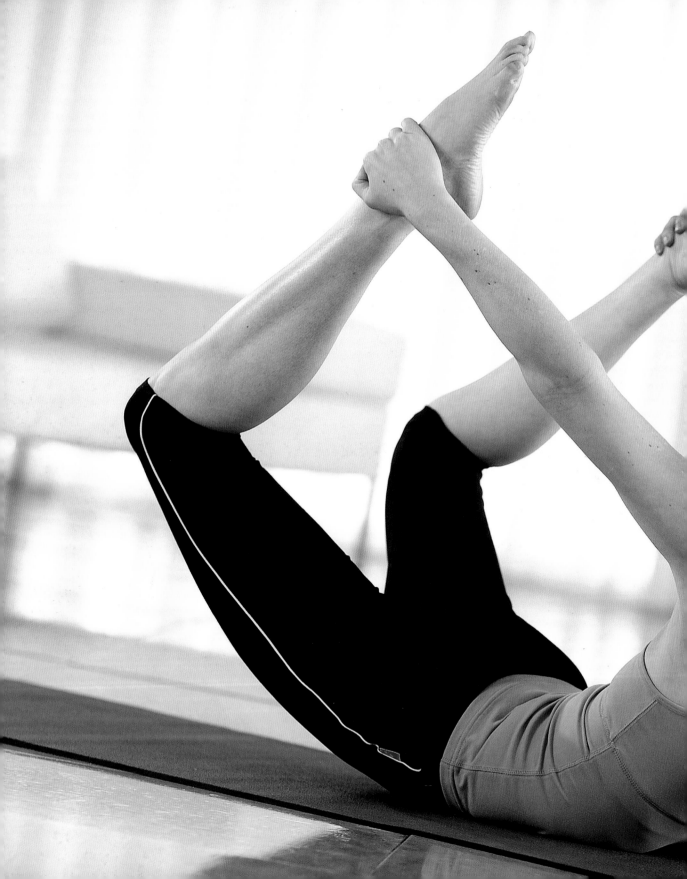

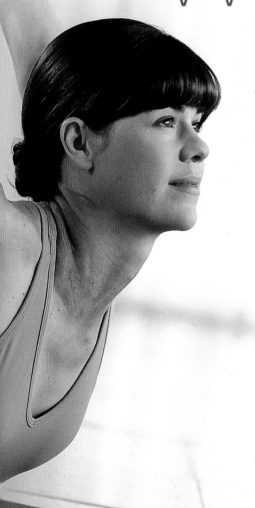
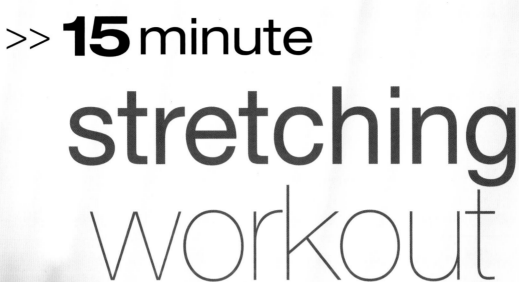

>> **15** minute

stretching
workout

Suzanne Martin P.T., D.P.T

>> **defining** the stretch

Welcome to the world of stretching. Not only will you learn how to stretch properly, but you will also find many types of stretches here. Forget all those preconceived notions about the value of holding a stretch for an indefinite amount of time. Let these stretches move you.

There's more than one way to stretch. That's because there's more to it than simply stretching muscles. Arteries, veins, and nerves that supply the muscles are involved, too. What is also important is the stretch of the fascia – the connective tissue that permeates the whole body, wraps around the muscles, and holds them close to the skeleton.

Think of it as biomechanical "architecture". The bones are the scaffolding and the fascia is the bricks and mortar that support the volume of the structure. The fascia adapts to its environment. If you were put into a small cupboard and made to sit in a crouched position for days on end, over time your body would attempt to shrink to fit into the extreme environment. The fascia does the same.

Compensating for bad habits

Our bodies are remarkably forgiving because we still function, even with poor posture – rounded shoulders and a forward head, or a protruding belly or collapsing ankles. The body compensates for weaknesses or faulty habits, but the compensations become "solidified", altering the patterns of our fascia and muscles. For this reason, we need different types of stretching to reverse any tightening to which our body has become accustomed.

Stretching strategies

We also need different stretches to address the properties of the various parts of our body. Moving stretches where, for instance, the head is rotating, the knee is bending, or the arm is circling, tend to

> ## >> **types** of stretching
>
> - **Re-coordination stretches** increase range by changing repetitive motor patterns caused by right or left dominance.
> - **Reciprocal stretches** use the natural shortening and lengthening effect on either side of a joint to create more stretch.
> - **Fascial stretches** focus on the fascia and help to balance muscle connections; they are particularly effective for opening and stretching the torso.

be re-coordination stretches. They help to break up the body patterns we develop from being right- or left-handed, as well the patterns that come from other re-occurring motions. Merely changing the direction of those familiar patterns can significantly increase our range of motion.

Another stretching strategy has to do with stretching muscles on the opposite side of joints. This is called reciprocal stretching. For instance, when you bend your elbow, the muscles on the front side of the joint – the biceps – shorten, and those on the other side – the triceps – have to lengthen to allow the motion. Using reciprocal stretching techniques automatically relaxes the lengthening side, allowing those muscles to stretch.

Stretching the fascia

Other types of stretches work on stretching the fascia in several ways. Stretching the spine using a breathing and rippling action helps to stretch the torso from horizontal segment to horizontal segment. Another fascial stretch works on stretching the muscle connection chain that runs from the waist, down the back of the leg, and into the foot (see pp.14–15). This programme also includes some stretches specifically designed to glide the arm and leg nerves in their sheaths, which allows greater ease of motion. The details make the difference; read the instructions carefully to find the precision that will give you your best stretch.

The devil's in the detail. Find the precision you need for each stretch by studying the demonstrations and imagining the cues.

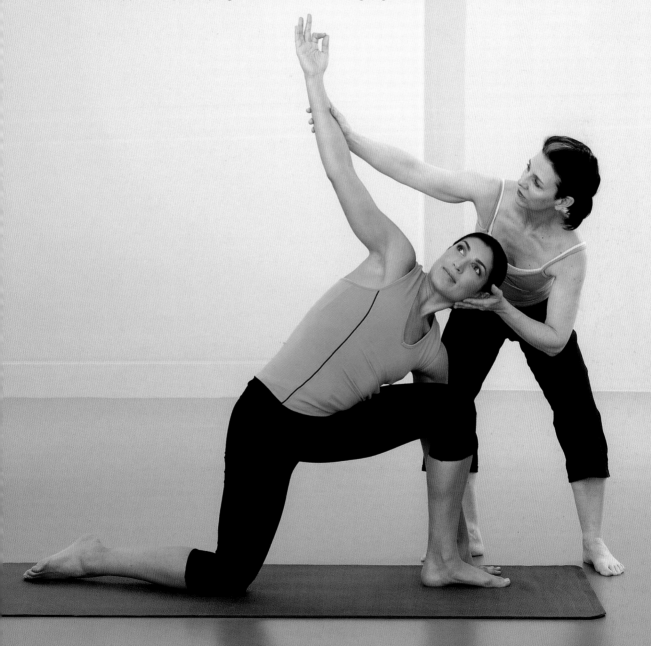

>> **muscle** connections

Proper positioning of the arms, legs, and head helps us to physically find the link between muscle and connective tissue. Using focus and intent when we line these extremities up with the torso gives us a powerful tool for changing body posture and developing flexibility.

The science of biomechanics identifies various structural body connections and physical forces that are involved in body function. In order to devise appropriate exercises, it is necessary to use our knowledge of the nature of our body parts (how plastic, or changeable, the various components are) to create the effect we need. Three important structural connections in the body that we have to consider are the "X" model, the inner unit, and the lateral system.

The "X" model
The "X" model shows the connection between what is going on externally and the inner unit (see below). It shows how the limbs are connected with each other and how these connections pass right through the inner unit. Think deep; think three-dimensional. The right arm, for example, is connected to the left leg and vice versa. The positioning of the head, which can weigh up to 6.8kg (15lb), is also important. Tipping it in any direction activates an intricate system of overlapping muscles that both bind the head into the trunk and yet allow a marvellous telescoping range to the neck.

The inner unit
Various groups of muscles form the inner unit. These are the muscles at the bottom of the torso (the pelvic floor), the deep abdominal muscles, the transverse abdominals at the sides of the abdomen, the deep low-back muscles, the multifidi (a group

> ### >> **pulling it all** together
>
> - **Coordination** between opposing limbs and the trunk is demonstrated by the "X" model concept.
> - **Precision** in stretching is created by achieving stabilization of the inner unit, which provides a firm foundation.
> - **Elongation of the lateral system** promotes symmetry and balance.

of muscles either side of the spine), and the muscles deep inside the rib cage (the diaphragm).

Working the muscles of the inner unit correctly – with good form – promotes low-back and pelvic health. The exercise instructions also help you to use the inner unit as a stabilizing foundation, giving more precision when you stretch the external parts.

The lateral system
The lateral system connects the muscles and fascia (see p.12) that run down the sides of the body. Think of it as a long road running from the triceps in the upper arm, past the armpit, down the side of the ribs and waist, extending down the side of the leg past the thigh and shin, and ending at the side of the foot. This lateral system is often overlooked, but opening it through stretching is key to balancing the body and improving posture.

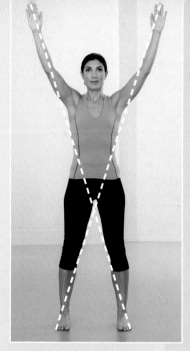

The **"X" model** shows the link between what goes on internally and externally. Opposite sides of the body criss-cross, attaching the limbs and head to the torso.

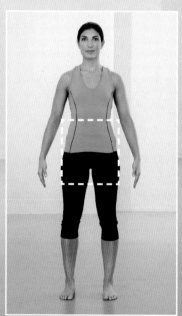

The **inner unit** is the foundation of our body. It houses our centre of gravity. Anchoring this area provides a counterbalance to, and increased effectiveness for, each stretch.

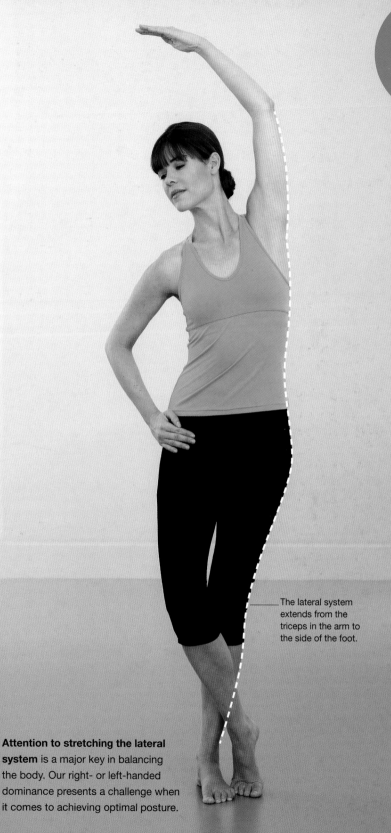

The lateral system extends from the triceps in the arm to the side of the foot.

Attention to stretching the lateral system is a major key in balancing the body. Our right- or left-handed dominance presents a challenge when it comes to achieving optimal posture.

>> **flexibility** and posture

Genetics dictate how flexible you are and also your postural body type. Stiffness and over-flexibility both cause aches, pains, and difficulty in day-to-day activities. Explore your flexibility with these easy tests, and strive to find your best neutral posture.

Gravity has a greater impact upon our posture when we are upright in sitting or standing. If we give in to it, the "segments" of our body collapse (see below left). The result is that our muscles are out of balance and our joints are misaligned.

Stretching counterbalances this and helps you develop a good neutral posture. You start by using good form and working the muscles of the inner unit (see p.14). This helps you stretch the chest and shorten the upper-back muscles, open the lower back and engage the abs, as well as stretch the front of the hips and thighs, and the calves.

Practising sitting and standing tall also solidifies your intent to push vertically upwards against the force of gravity. The beauty of this formula is that it applies to all body types and levels of flexibility.

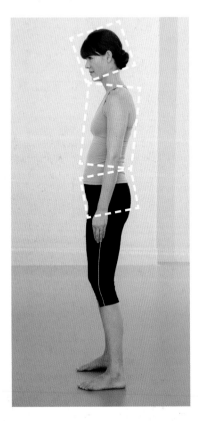
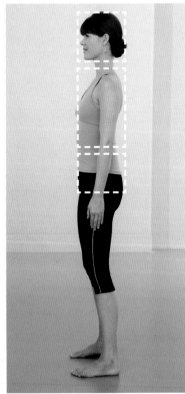

Gravity breaks us into unbalanced segments (far left). The head falls forward. The chest shortens and sinks, and the upper back rounds. The lower back tightens and collapses, and the abdomen protrudes. The front of the thighs and hips tighten, while the hip extensors slacken. Body weight lists back on the heels, shortening the calves.

The goal is to balance the segments and achieve neutral posture, with a straight line running from the head through the pelvis (left). Note especially how the weight of the heavy head is now balanced directly over the pelvis, which houses our centre of gravity. This alignment puts the least amount of strain on the spine as well as on the other joints in the body.

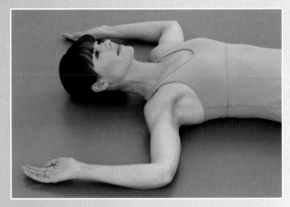

Test the mobility of your shoulders and upper back. Lie on the floor with your arms bent and your forearms parallel with the sides of you head. Your muscles are over-tight if your head and forearms do not touch the floor.

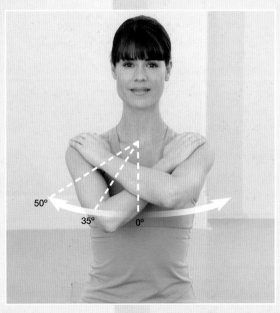

Test the mobility of your spine, rib cage and neck. From a seated position, cross your arms, put each hand on the opposite shoulder and rotate your torso. Note how far you can go. Anything less than 35° indicates that your muscles are over-tight. Being right-handed or left-handed affects how far you can rotate.

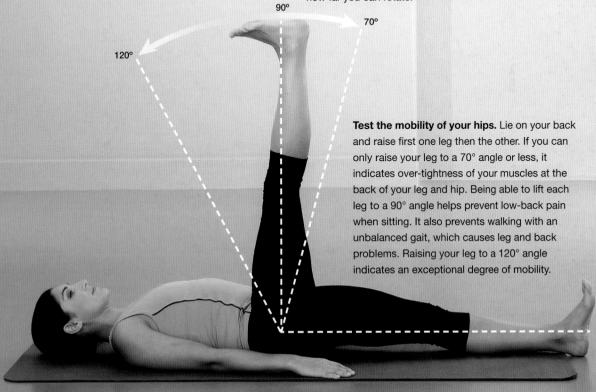

Test the mobility of your hips. Lie on your back and raise first one leg then the other. If you can only raise your leg to a 70° angle or less, it indicates over-tightness of your muscles at the back of your leg and hip. Being able to lift each leg to a 90° angle helps prevent low-back pain when sitting. It also prevents walking with an unbalanced gait, which causes leg and back problems. Raising your leg to a 120° angle indicates an exceptional degree of mobility.

>> **imagery** as a tool

Use imagery as a tool to help create precision and a sense of the inner layers of your body in your stretches. Connecting everyday concepts to the exercises gives your stretches an effective edge. Strive to internalize the cues. They are the key to true physical transformation.

Actors, musicians, and dancers use imagery to help them "act out" their message. Children play imaginary roles in imaginary settings to prepare for adult life. As adults, we can employ visualization to help us make our exercise more effective.

The programmes in this book contain some imagery cues that ask you to use your imagination. Focus on them to help coordinate your muscles and access the deeper connections of your body. For example, "Lift the imaginary swimming-pool water" asks you to press upwards in the abdomen when you're lying on your front. Mention of "smile lines" is a cue for you to hold your hips in true extension when lying down, and gives you the range of motion you need to achieve a neutral pelvis. When you get it right, two arcs separate the buttocks from the upper thighs or hamstrings (see below).

By training these deeper muscles to engage as you perform your stretching exercises, you also train them to engage when you carry out your everyday activities. Although some images apply to certain body positions, such as finding the smile lines while lying on your front, you can also relate to them in other positions. In other words, you can find your smile lines when you're standing, too. They can help you find your neutral posture (see p.16).

The imagery I use is truly the key to taking your exercise life into your daily life. Study the pictures in the exercises on these two pages, and start a lifelong habit of using your body more completely.

Imagining water pushing up against your abdomen deepens abdominal connections. Visualizing "smile lines" stabilizes your pelvis and brings precision to hip stretches.

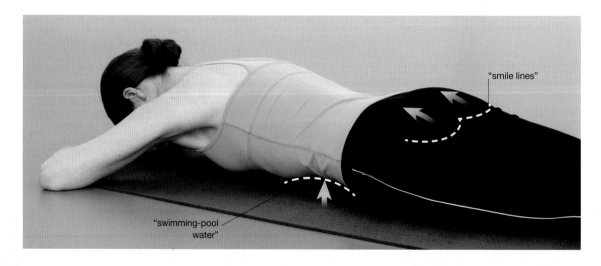

"smile lines"

"swimming-pool water"

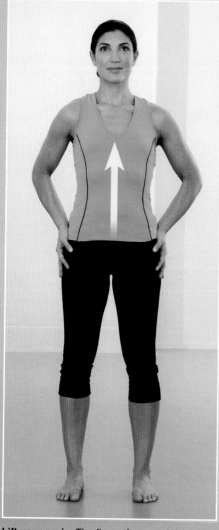

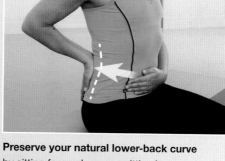

Preserve your natural lower-back curve by sitting forward on your sitting bones. Simultaneously pull your navel to your spine to sandwich your waist with a corset of muscles.

Coordinate the stretch between your head and legs. Reach your head out of your collarbones, like a turtle reaching its head out of its shell. At the same time, balance and reach out through your top foot.

Lift your groin. The floor of your pelvis should be buoyed upwards, just as a parachute fills with air. Feel the movement, like a lift ascending up your spine towards your head.

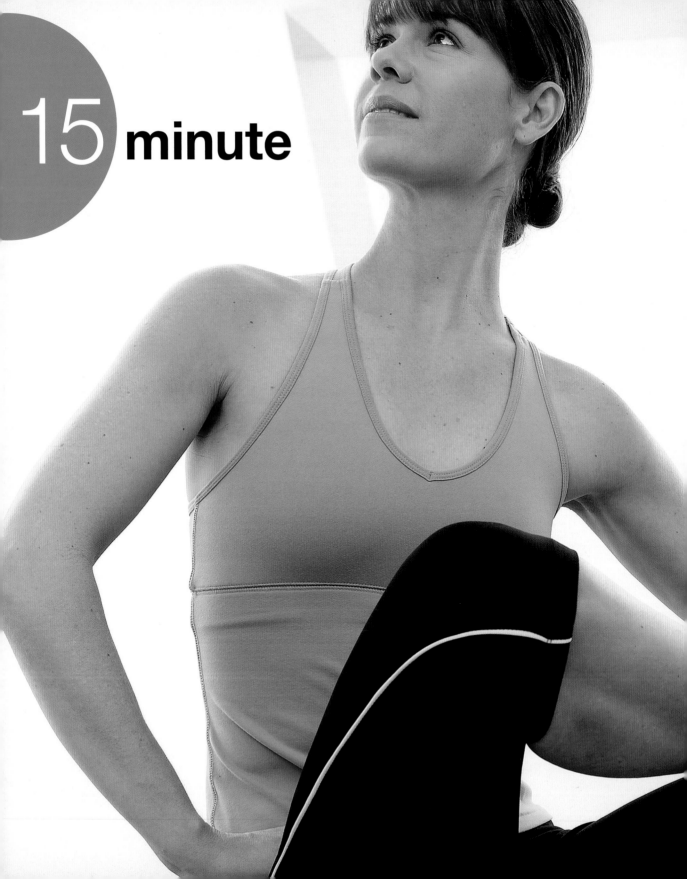

15 minute

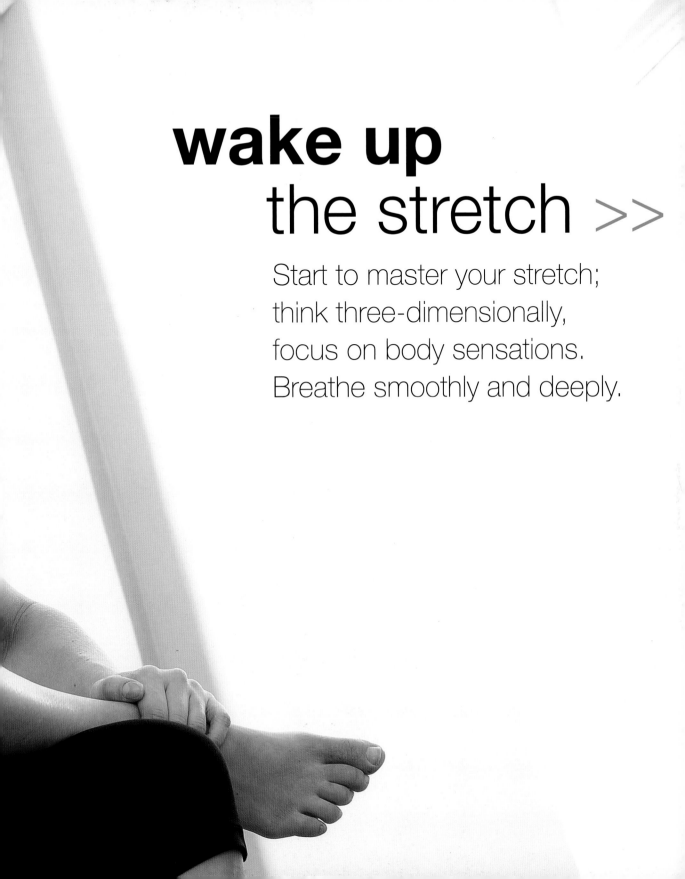

wake up
the stretch >>

Start to master your stretch;
think three-dimensionally,
focus on body sensations.
Breathe smoothly and deeply.

>> **wake up** the stretch

Your stretch journey starts with a sequence that creates suppleness and wakes up your stretch. No matter what your level, as you stretch your whole body, you'll find the fluid motion of this sequence as slinky as a long cat yawn. Try to imagine that you're "joining the dots" as you weave your way through each and every movement.

Stretching is a skill that everyone can master. This sequence emphasizes the various techniques you'll need and the sensory elements of stretch that together will help to make your stretch possible. Being able to identify muscle tone is a crucial first step. Next, learning to stabilize one part of the body while another moves away from the stabilizing part is key to the effectiveness of a lengthening stretch. Breathing into tight body areas such as the back of the rib cage demands discipline and focus. Loosening and circling motions help to oil the joints and loosen restrictive connective tissue, thus prompting muscles to expand and contract. Re-coordination exercises (see p.12) make new ranges of motion a possibility for everyone.

The exercises

Feel as much of your body as you can in the Hand pull. Memorize this muscular feeling and strive to carry that feeling into the rest of the sequence. Make the Elbow circles as sensory and luscious as if you were moving through a pool of honey. Direct the flow of your breath very specifically into any tight parts of the diaphragm. This exercise may feel difficult at first, but it can give you a very satisfying sense of relaxation.

The seated exercises may seem easy, but use the surface and structure of the chair to explore your orientation in space. Notice the relationship of your hip, rib, head, arm, and leg placements.

> ## >> **tips for** wake up the stretch
>
> - **Internalize your stretches** by giving as much detailed focus to your body sensations as possible.
>
> - **Try to imagine** the infrastructure – the skeletal part that is moving – such as your arms moving against your upper torso.
>
> - **Work to identify** which parts are anchoring and which parts are moving.
>
> - **Strive to feel the entire path of the motion**, not just the end points.
>
> - **Breathe in long, flowing, time-released breaths**, as suggested by the guide music; be sure not to hold your breath.

The physical boundary of the chair not only provides landmarks so you can judge how far a stretch is moving, it can also give you a sense of where your deep muscles are, which can help if you feel your movement is restricted. Sitting on a firm surface is also a sneaky way to feel some input up into your sitting bones. This pressure gives a neurological stimulus to your "righting" reflex, which helps you to lengthen up against gravity.

The Seated cross-leg twist and Shoulder wedge also show you how to press one body part against another to increase the stretch, as well as adding a strengthening element to your stretches.

At the other end of the scale are the Shoulder ovals. They demonstrate an instance where learning to respect a joint's boundary is of great importance, since neck, arms, and shoulders tend to be more sensitive to injury thanks to their potential for extreme movement. The Shoulder ovals also provide a superb nerve stretch and glide – a nerve glide being a movement that creates frictionless motion of the nerve. This, ultimately, will increase the range of movement of the whole of your upper body.

Simple stretching positions while sitting can bring about big changes when you perform them with coordination, precision, and intent.

>> **hand pull**

1 Stand with your hands by your hips, feet just past shoulder-width apart, and toes firmly planted into the floor. Feel as if your legs are pressing outwards. Lift your groin muscles towards the head (see p.19) and firm your hips. Slowly exhale as you open your arms to the sides, turning your palms forward.

2 Clasp your hands overhead in an "O" shape, then pull on the hands as if you are trying to pull them apart. Feel as if you are pulling your hands and feet away from each other as you take 2 long breaths. Keep the shape as you exhale and relax for 2 more breaths. Repeat the pull, then relax.

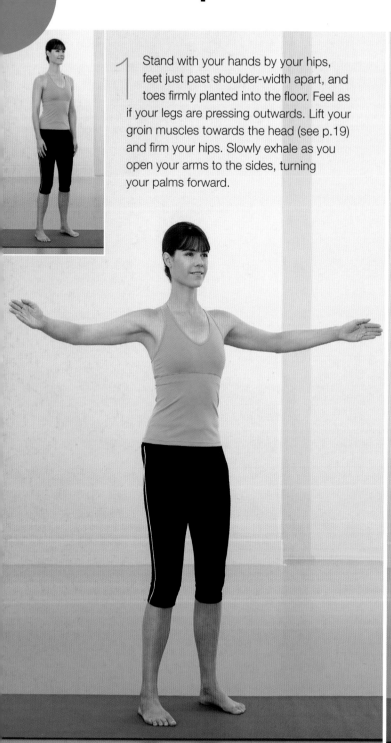

pull

feel it here

push apart

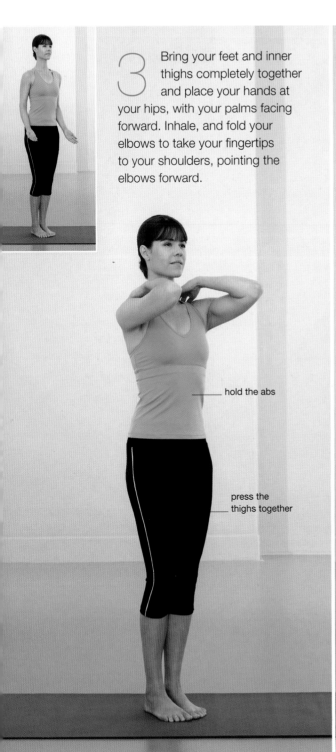

3 Bring your feet and inner thighs completely together and place your hands at your hips, with your palms facing forward. Inhale, and fold your elbows to take your fingertips to your shoulders, pointing the elbows forward.

hold the abs

press the thighs together

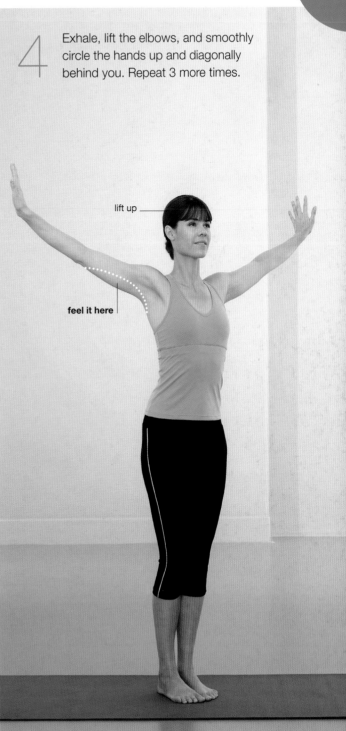

4 Exhale, lift the elbows, and smoothly circle the hands up and diagonally behind you. Repeat 3 more times.

lift up

feel it here

>> rib breath

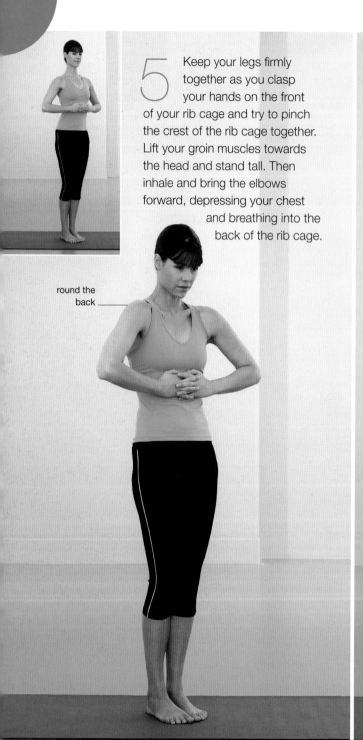

5 Keep your legs firmly together as you clasp your hands on the front of your rib cage and try to pinch the crest of the rib cage together. Lift your groin muscles towards the head and stand tall. Then inhale and bring the elbows forward, depressing your chest and breathing into the back of the rib cage.

round the back

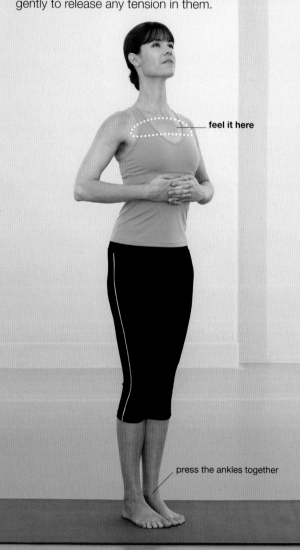

6 Reverse the movement. Exhale, open the chest, lengthen up through your head, and look diagonally upwards. Allow your elbows to come backwards. Repeat 2 more times, inhaling as you bring the elbows forward, and exhaling as you open the chest. Release your hands and shake them gently to release any tension in them.

feel it here

press the ankles together

>> **side reach**

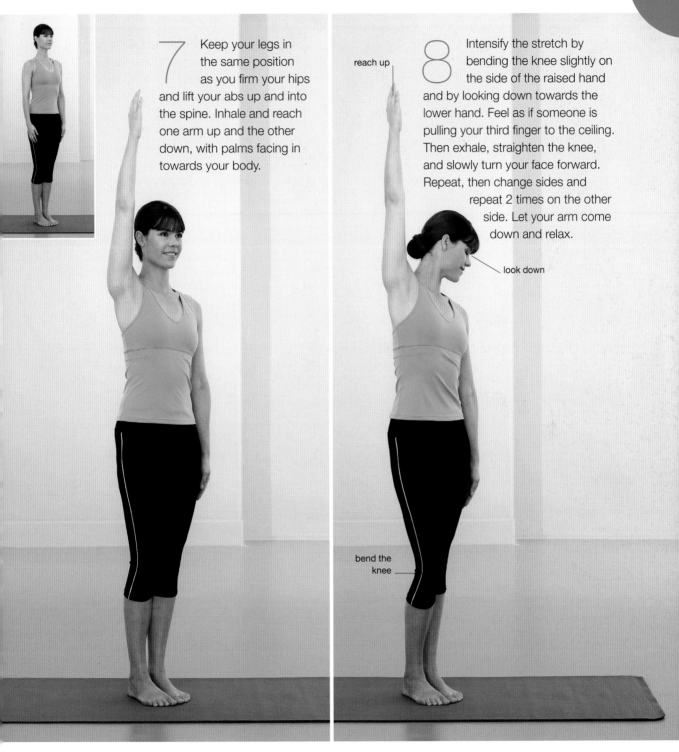

7 Keep your legs in the same position as you firm your hips and lift your abs up and into the spine. Inhale and reach one arm up and the other down, with palms facing in towards your body.

reach up

8 Intensify the stretch by bending the knee slightly on the side of the raised hand and by looking down towards the lower hand. Feel as if someone is pulling your third finger to the ceiling. Then exhale, straighten the knee, and slowly turn your face forward. Repeat, then change sides and repeat 2 times on the other side. Let your arm come down and relax.

look down

bend the knee

>> lift & bow

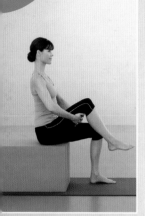

9 Sit on the edge of a chair with your feet hip-width apart. Feel your sitting bones pressing equally on the seat. Sit tall, lift your groin muscles towards your head, then hold onto one thigh and lift the knee towards the ceiling. Inhale, then lift up into your waist and bow your head towards your knee.

10 Exhale and reverse, lifting your chest and face diagonally up towards the ceiling. Repeat 2 more times, inhaling as you bow, and exhaling as you lift. Lower the foot to the floor and repeat on the other side.

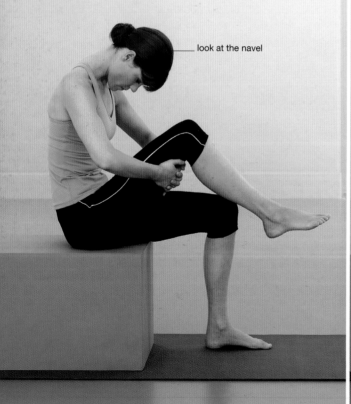

look at the navel

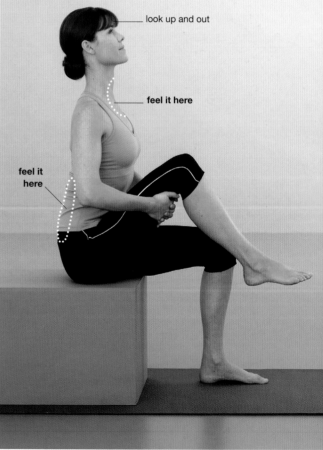

look up and out

feel it here

feel it here

11 Remain sitting towards the edge of your seat. Extend one foot out on the floor in front of you, keeping the knee a little bent, and pressing the sole and big toe of the foot firmly on the floor. Place your hands on the same thigh. Inhale as you round your back.

12 Exhale and reverse the curve. Start from the lower back, and move through the middle and upper back with a ripple effect to lift the chest and face diagonally towards the ceiling. Inhale, round, and repeat, then repeat the whole stretch on the other side. Roll your shoulders and release.

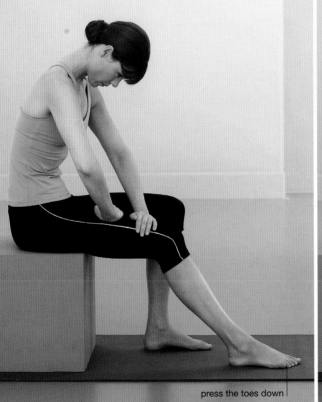

press the toes down

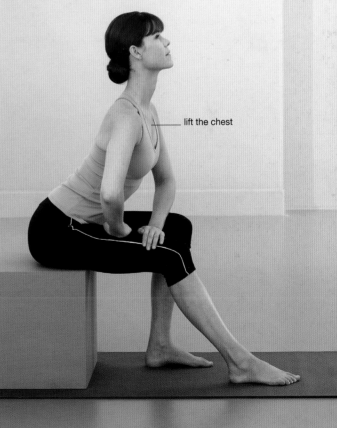

lift the chest

>> **seated cross-leg twist**

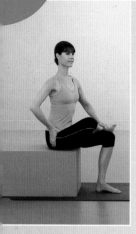

13 Remain seated, cross one foot on top of the opposite thigh, and hold onto your ankle with the other hand. Place the same hand as your crossed leg on your hip. Inhale, lift your groin muscles towards the head, lengthen your spine, and bow your head towards your knee.

14 Exhale, lift your chest, and turn your torso towards your crossed leg. Look past your shoulder. Repeat 2 more times, inhaling as you bow and exhaling as you lift, then repeat 3 times on the other side. Slowly release the leg, come out of the position, and gently move your back to release any tension.

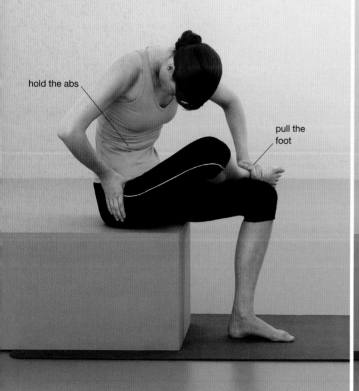

hold the abs

pull the foot

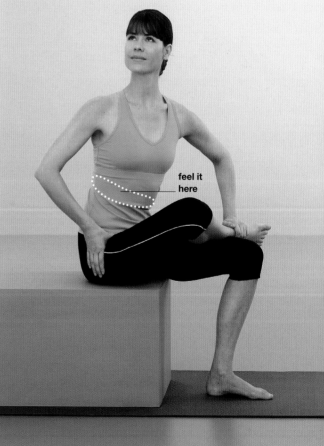

feel it here

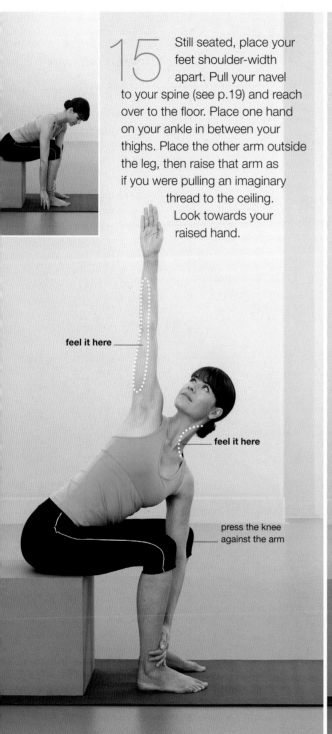

15 Still seated, place your feet shoulder-width apart. Pull your navel to your spine (see p.19) and reach over to the floor. Place one hand on your ankle in between your thighs. Place the other arm outside the leg, then raise that arm as if you were pulling an imaginary thread to the ceiling. Look towards your raised hand.

feel it here

feel it here

press the knee against the arm

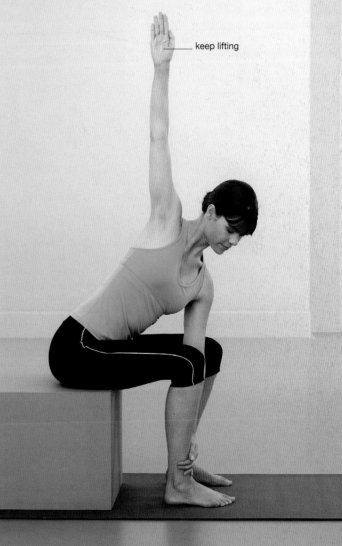

16 Exhale, keep your arm lifted, and consciously rotate your neck as you look down. Repeat 2 more times, inhaling as you look up, and exhaling as you look down. Bring the arm down and repeat 3 times on the other side. Roll to sit up. Take a deep breath, and relax.

keep lifting

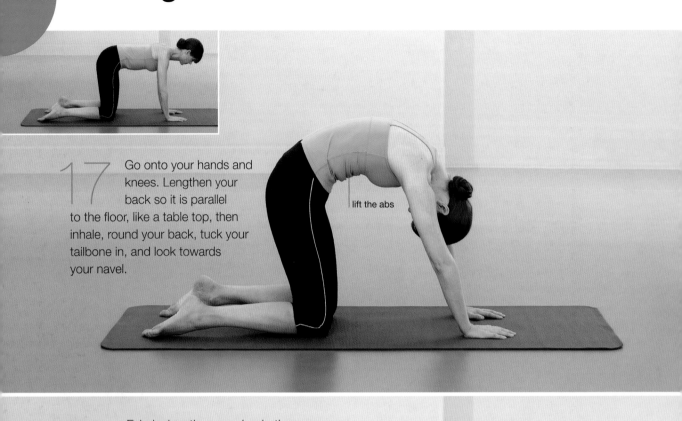

17 Go onto your hands and knees. Lengthen your back so it is parallel to the floor, like a table top, then inhale, round your back, tuck your tailbone in, and look towards your navel.

lift the abs

18 Exhale, lengthen your back, then sway your hips and head towards each other. Repeat on the other side, always inhaling as you round your back and exhaling as you take your hips and head towards each other. Repeat 1 more time each side.

sway the hips towards the face

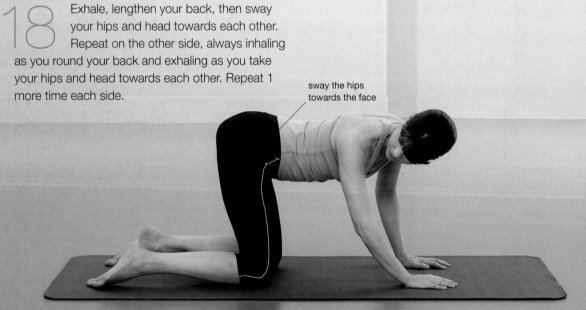

>> **arm fans**

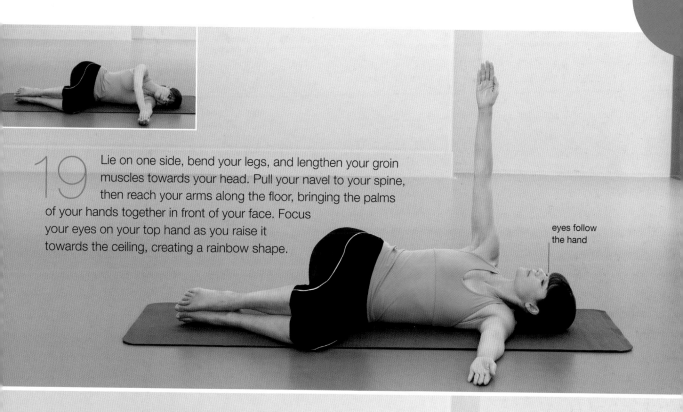

19 Lie on one side, bend your legs, and lengthen your groin muscles towards your head. Pull your navel to your spine, then reach your arms along the floor, bringing the palms of your hands together in front of your face. Focus your eyes on your top hand as you raise it towards the ceiling, creating a rainbow shape.

eyes follow the hand

20 Continue moving the arm and reach behind you to the floor, allowing your shoulders and torso to rotate with the arm. Try not to move your knees. Exhale, then reach up with the hand as you reverse, "painting the ceiling" with your fingertips until your hands are together again. Repeat 2 more times, inhaling as you open the arm, exhaling as you bring the palms together again. Roll over to the other side and repeat.

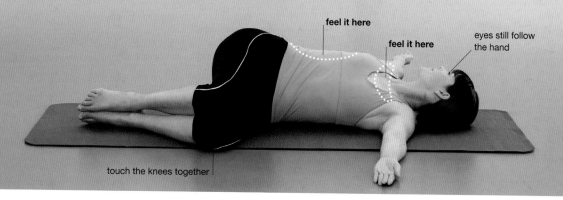

feel it here

feel it here

eyes still follow the hand

touch the knees together

>> modified cobra

21 Go onto your stomach, firm and tighten your hips, and feel the smile lines (see p.18) between your glutes and your hamstrings. Lift the groin muscles towards the head. Feel the imaginary swimming-pool water lifting your abdomen off the floor (see p.18). Reach your hands out onto the floor in front of you.

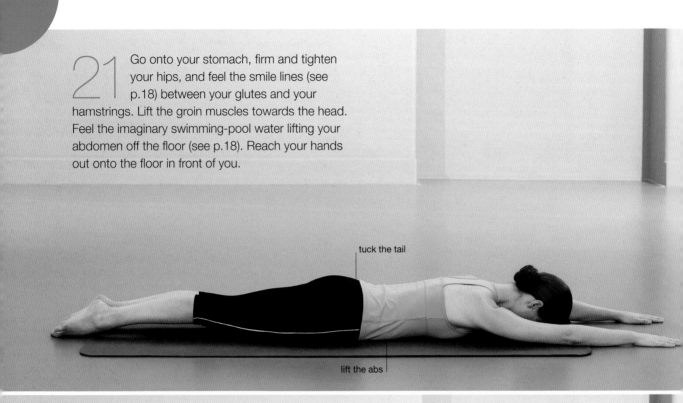

tuck the tail

lift the abs

22 Inhale as you drag your hands along the floor towards your shoulders, keeping the abdomen tight and lifting your front body so your ribs come off the floor. Exhale, slide the arms out in front of you, and take your face back to the floor. Repeat, then relax and breathe normally.

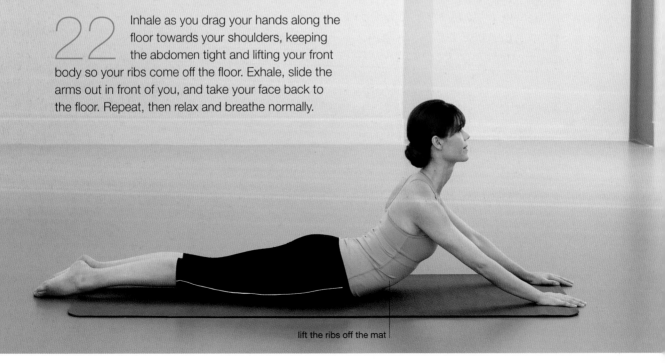

lift the ribs off the mat

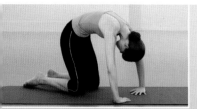

23 Tighten the waist, lift the hips, and come up to a perfect hands and knees position. Point the fingers of the hands in towards each other, then inhale and reach one shoulder down towards the opposite hand.

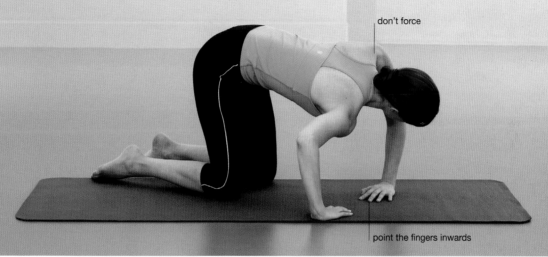

don't force

point the fingers inwards

24 Sweep the chest across the floor, past centre towards the other hand, then exhale and continue circling in the same direction as you round your back. Your shoulders should be describing an oval in space. Keep going in the same direction for 2 more ovals, then change direction and reverse for 2 more ovals.

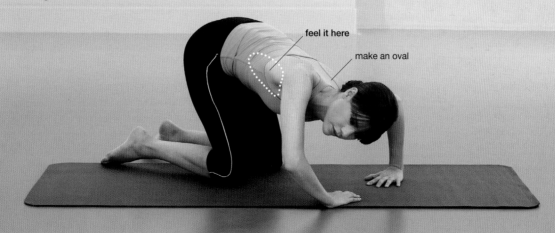

feel it here

make an oval

wake up the stretch >>

wake up the stretch at a glance

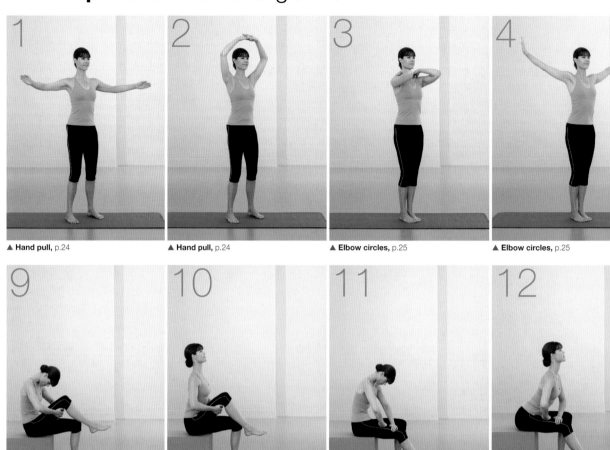

▲ Hand pull, p.24

▲ Hand pull, p.24

▲ Elbow circles, p.25

▲ Elbow circles, p.25

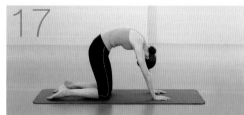

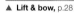

▲ Lift & bow, p.28

▲ Lift & bow, p.28

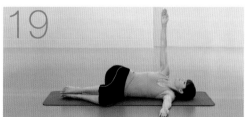

▲ Seated cat, p.29

▲ Seated cat, p.29

▲ Alligator/
cat, p.32

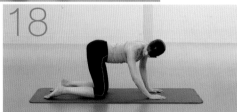

▲ Alligator/cat, p.32

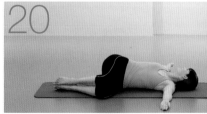

▲ Arm fans,
p.33

▲ Arm fans, p.33

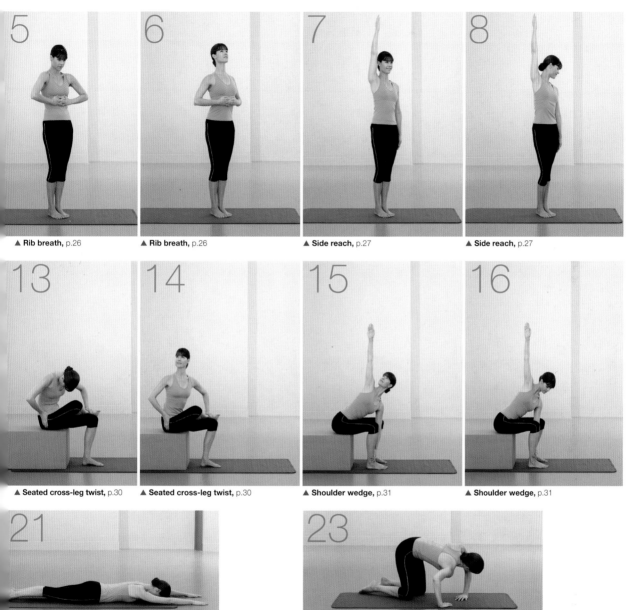

5 ▲ Rib breath, p.26

6 ▲ Rib breath, p.26

7 ▲ Side reach, p.27

8 ▲ Side reach, p.27

13 ▲ Seated cross-leg twist, p.30

14 ▲ Seated cross-leg twist, p.30

15 ▲ Shoulder wedge, p.31

16 ▲ Shoulder wedge, p.31

21 ▲ Modified cobra, p.34

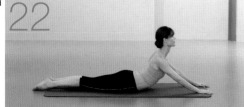

22 ▲ Modified cobra, p.34

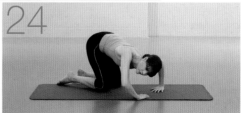

23 ▲ Shoulder ovals p.35

24 ▲ Shoulder ovals, p.35

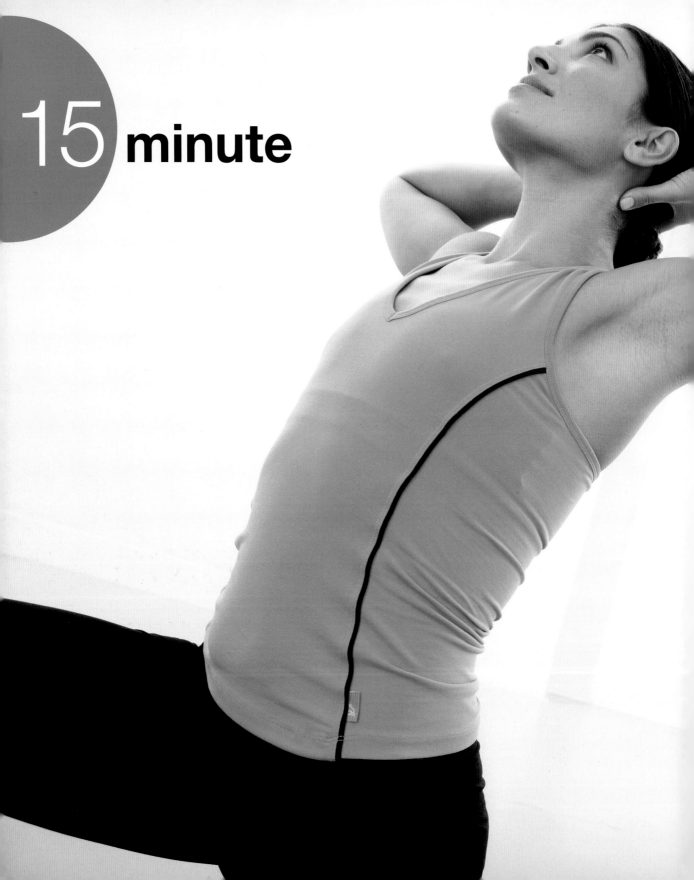

15 minute

posture stretch >>

Find your centre.
Elongate your waist;
extend up against
the force of gravity.

>> **posture** stretch

We all want healthy posture. Although we live in an imperfect world, nearly perfect posture can be achieved by methodically balancing our body against gravity's pull. Where the body leads, the mind goes. Improving posture will lift your outlook on life as well as giving you confidence and endurance against everyday stresses.

Stretching for healthy posture means fighting against the pull of gravity. If we do not work against gravity's pull, then the longer we live, the more bent and deformed we become. A typical gravitational pull creates a forward-jutting chin, a tight chest, and rounded shoulders. Carrying on down the body, the abdomen becomes lax and the lower back becomes tighter. A domino effect continues on into the legs, shortening the front of the thighs and creating a loose area around the glutes. The end-result is an off-centre line, with tight calves causing the body weight to fall back into the heels (see p.16). It's no wonder joints wear out before their time. We're all living longer, so our joints – which are a key factor in our quality of life – are important to us. The value of healthy posture cannot be stressed too much. Not only do we achieve a pleasing cosmetic effect by standing upright, we also increase our vitality, since standing well promotes optimal lung capacity, which provides more oxygen for the brain to function well.

The exercises
The Posture stretch sequence follows a muscle-balancing formula as well as reinforcing the neuro-developmental sequence – in other words, the basic movement patterns that get a baby from lying down to standing and walking. The Posture stretch sequence uses all the positions that babies must achieve on their journey to walking.

> ## >> **tips for** posture stretch
>
> - **Focus on the ultimate goal** of elongating your entire body in every exercise.
>
> - **Notice how each exercise builds** towards firm, upright posture.
>
> - **Modify when needed**. Be sensible and use extra padding under the knees if they are tender.
>
> - **Enhance balance** by focusing your eyes on a fixed object or by holding onto furniture, if necessary.
>
> - **In the final standing exercise**, focus first on stretching out and elongating your waist as you lengthen your ribs up and off the pelvis; locate your head weight over the centre of gravity in the pelvic bowl.

Starting with exercises lying on the back, trunk control is developed which enables optimum control of the limbs. Pay special attention to the various parts of the front of the trunk in the Elongations. Notice how the "W's" exercise straightens and elongates you, combating the typical foetal curling position many adopt when asleep. Next, the Hurdler lat stretch balances both sides of the back of the waist. The Balance point stretch literally pushes the trunk and head up against gravity. Most of us don't notice how our back is pulling us down because our legs compensate, taking up most of the slack in the system. The Sidelying waist stretch stretches the deep muscles we use to stand and walk; be sure to pull the abdomen strongly up and into the spine to get the most benefit from this intense twist.

Progressing to kneeling on both knees usually shows us how tight the front of our thighs and hips can be. The Lunge opener prepares the body for full standing and evens out our walking pattern so that it is not lop-sided. Squatting and then alternating the motion by reaching the hips upwards in the Round back squat gives balance and leg strength as well as stretch. The rolling-back motion of the Hanging stretch lets the body register the weight of the trunk and head above the waist. These body parts are heavy, and need to be placed precisely above the firm foundation of the lower body. Ending with a Top-to-toe stretch coalesces the whole body, helping you to stand tall against the ever-present force of gravity.

Kneeling positions help lengthen the front of your body, counteracting hip tightness from prolonged sitting and the slump and fatigue associated with prolonged standing.

>> **elongations**

1 Lie on your back, with your legs hip-width apart. Reach your arms beyond your head on the floor and clasp your hands. Inhale and stretch your hands and feet away from each other. Simultaneously press your low back and ribs against the floor.

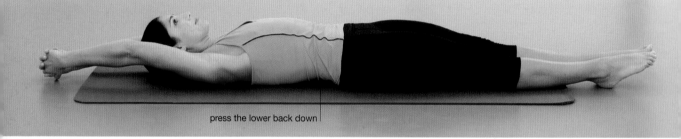

press the lower back down

2 Exhale as you relax, then inhale and stretch again. Finally, exhale and relax one more time.

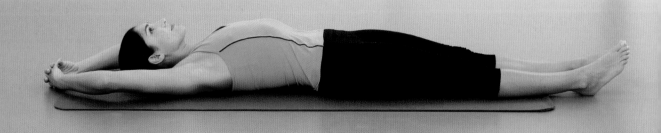

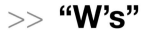

3 Stay on your back. Reach your arms out to the sides and bend your elbows to 90° with the backs of your hands and forearms towards the floor. If they don't touch the floor, don't force them. Inhale, then press the back of your head, forearms, shoulders, lower back, and thighs into the floor.

press the forearms down

4 Exhale and relax, releasing all the tension. Repeat by inhaling and pressing, and exhaling and releasing.

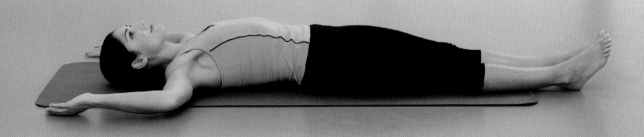

posture stretch >>

>> "C" stretch

5 Still lying on your back, reach your arms up beyond your head on the floor. Take one wrist and, keeping your shoulders against the floor, inhale and pull the wrist towards the opposite side, sliding your upper body slightly along the floor in the same direction.

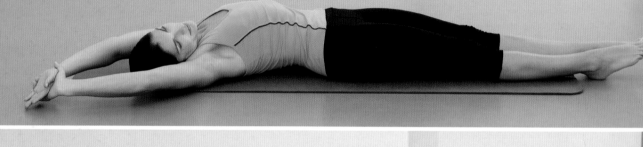

6 At the same time, cross the leg opposite the held wrist over the other leg, and slide your legs in the same direction. This adds an extra stretch and helps to make a letter "C" with your body. Stay, inhale, and tense your abdominal muscles, then exhale and lengthen into the "C". Hold for 4 breath cycles. Lengthen and release, move back to the centre, and repeat on the other side. Thump the thighs to release the lower back. Repeat on both sides, then thump the thighs one more time.

keep pulling
the wrist

pull the legs

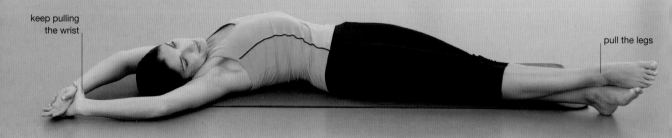

7 Remain on your back. Exhale, press your back against the floor, and slowly slide your feet towards your hips. Lift your feet, one at a time, and hold onto them from outside your legs, keeping your knees bent. If you can't reach your feet, hold onto your shins.

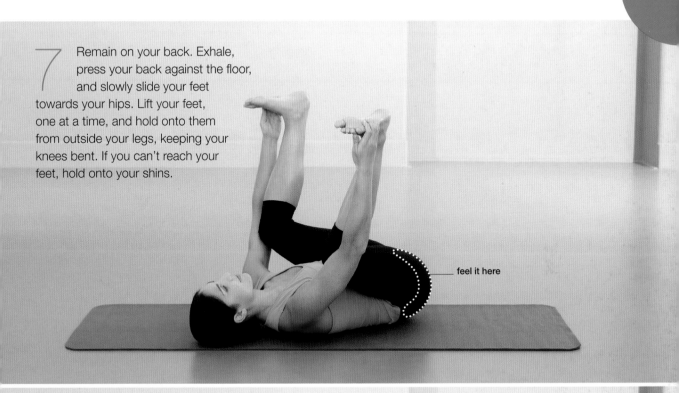

feel it here

8 Inhale, pull one knee down towards the floor, and rock towards that side. Then, exhale and release to return to centre. Repeat, rocking on the other side, then repeat for 2 more sets.

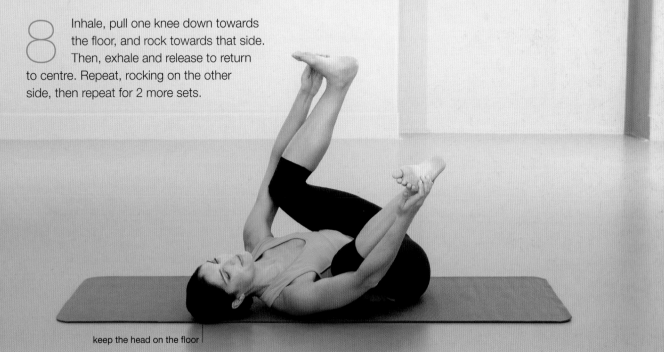

keep the head on the floor

>> **hurdler lat stretch**

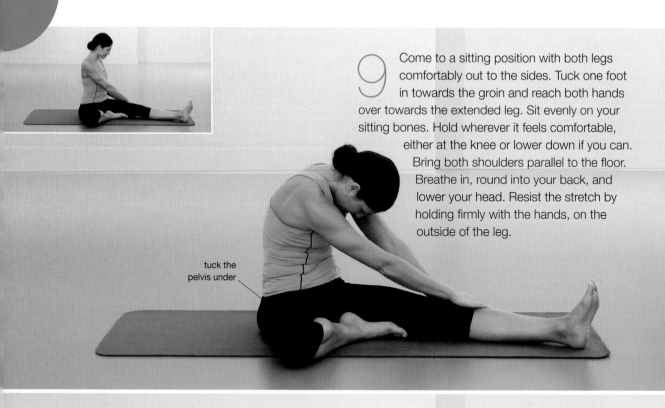

9 Come to a sitting position with both legs comfortably out to the sides. Tuck one foot in towards the groin and reach both hands over towards the extended leg. Sit evenly on your sitting bones. Hold wherever it feels comfortable, either at the knee or lower down if you can. Bring both shoulders parallel to the floor. Breathe in, round into your back, and lower your head. Resist the stretch by holding firmly with the hands, on the outside of the leg.

tuck the pelvis under

10 Exhale, pull forward with your hands, round the back even more, and look towards your navel. Repeat 2 more times, then release your hands, roll your shoulders, and repeat on the other side.

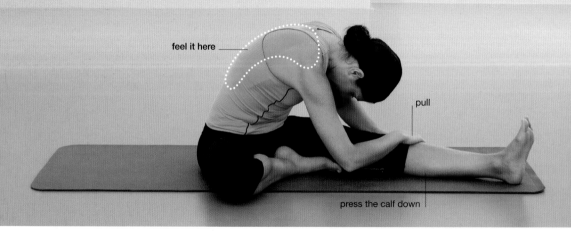

feel it here

pull

press the calf down

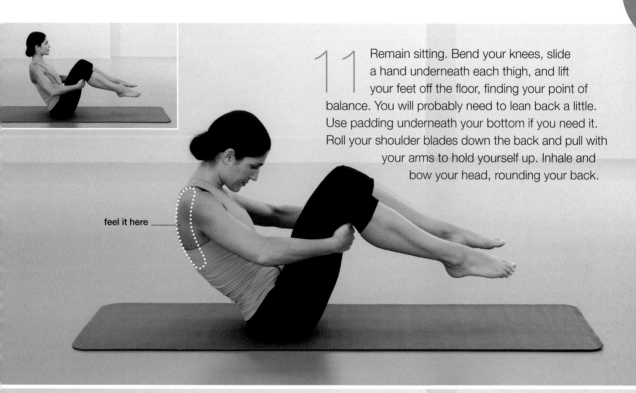

11 Remain sitting. Bend your knees, slide a hand underneath each thigh, and lift your feet off the floor, finding your point of balance. You will probably need to lean back a little. Use padding underneath your bottom if you need it. Roll your shoulder blades down the back and pull with your arms to hold yourself up. Inhale and bow your head, rounding your back.

feel it here

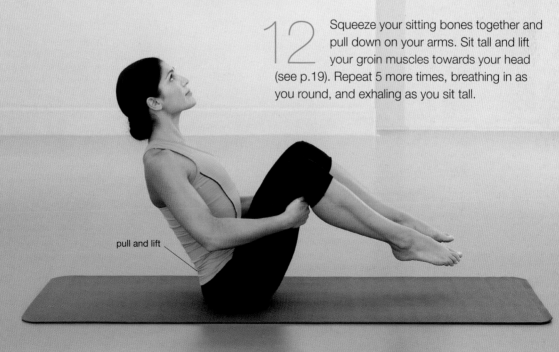

12 Squeeze your sitting bones together and pull down on your arms. Sit tall and lift your groin muscles towards your head (see p.19). Repeat 5 more times, breathing in as you round, and exhaling as you sit tall.

pull and lift

>> **sidelying waist stretch**

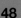

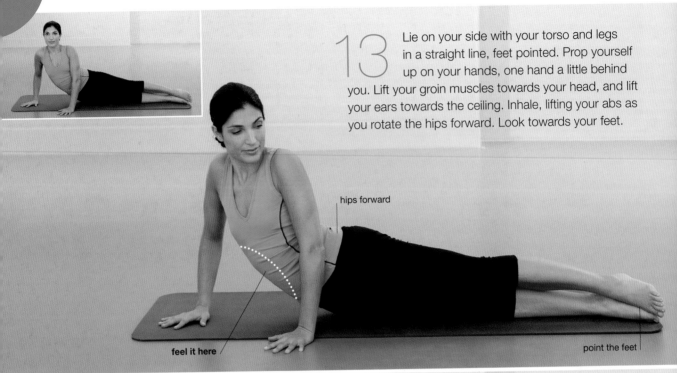

13 Lie on your side with your torso and legs in a straight line, feet pointed. Prop yourself up on your hands, one hand a little behind you. Lift your groin muscles towards your head, and lift your ears towards the ceiling. Inhale, lifting your abs as you rotate the hips forward. Look towards your feet.

hips forward

feel it here

point the feet

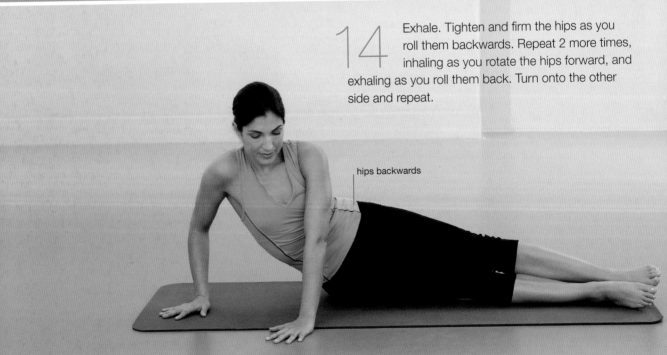

14 Exhale. Tighten and firm the hips as you roll them backwards. Repeat 2 more times, inhaling as you rotate the hips forward, and exhaling as you roll them back. Turn onto the other side and repeat.

hips backwards

>> **posture stretch**

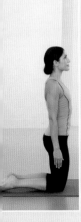

15 Kneel up, with your knees under your pelvis. Use padding underneath your knees if you need it. Tuck your pelvis under and press the hips forward. Find your smile lines (see p.18). Reach your arms behind you and clasp your hands behind your back, without over-arching the back. Inhale, press your hips together, and squeeze your glutes. Lift your chest and stretch your hands behind you.

16 Exhale, relax your hands and come back to centre. Repeat another 2 times.

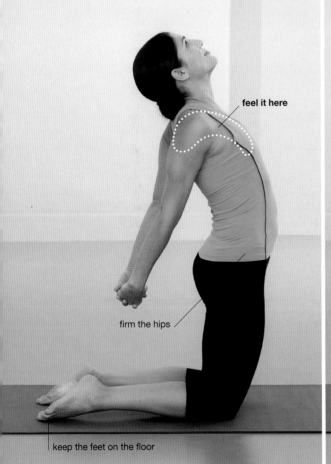

feel it here

firm the hips

keep the feet on the floor

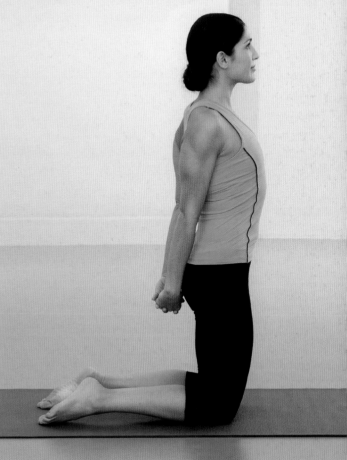

>> lunge opener

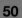

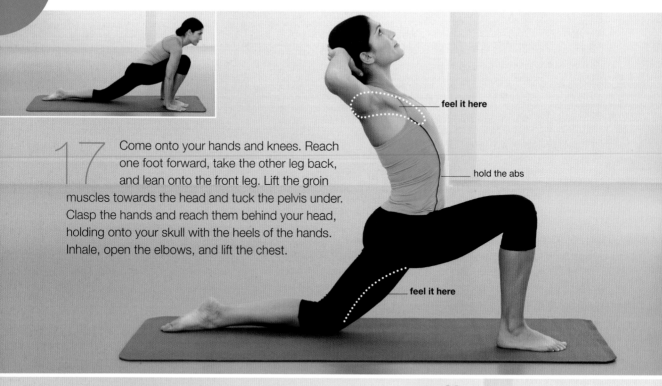

feel it here

hold the abs

feel it here

17 Come onto your hands and knees. Reach one foot forward, take the other leg back, and lean onto the front leg. Lift the groin muscles towards the head and tuck the pelvis under. Clasp the hands and reach them behind your head, holding onto your skull with the heels of the hands. Inhale, open the elbows, and lift the chest.

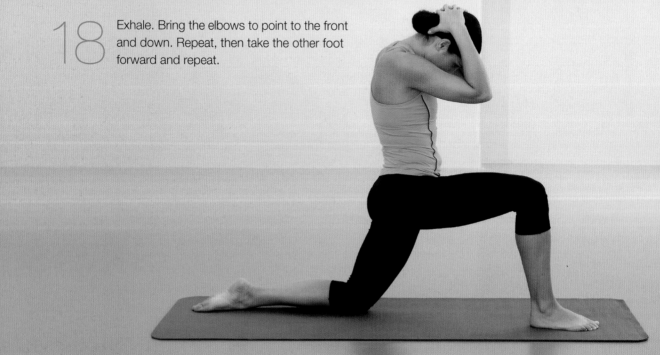

18 Exhale. Bring the elbows to point to the front and down. Repeat, then take the other foot forward and repeat.

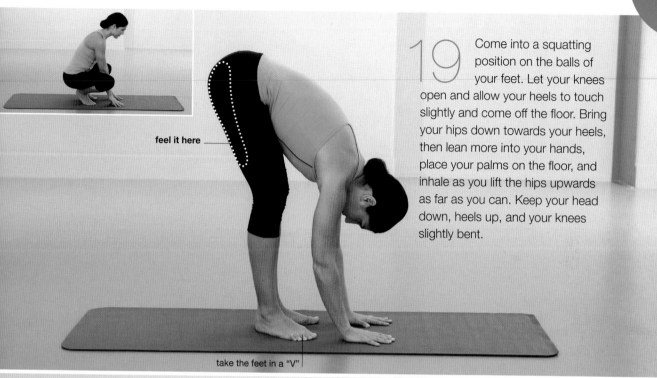

feel it here

take the feet in a "V"

19 Come into a squatting position on the balls of your feet. Let your knees open and allow your heels to touch slightly and come off the floor. Bring your hips down towards your heels, then lean more into your hands, place your palms on the floor, and inhale as you lift the hips upwards as far as you can. Keep your head down, heels up, and your knees slightly bent.

20 Take a long, slow exhalation as you round your back, tuck your hips in, and lower them towards the heels again, still keeping your head down. Repeat 2 more times.

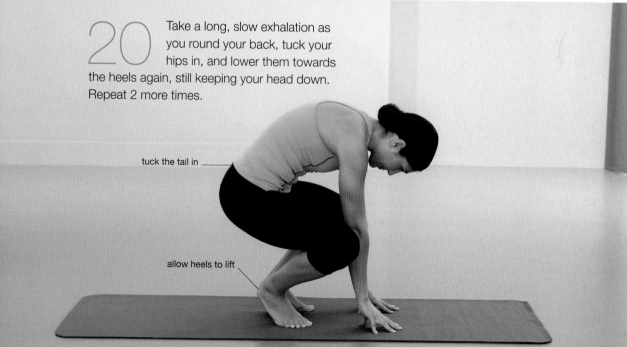

tuck the tail in

allow heels to lift

>> hanging stretch

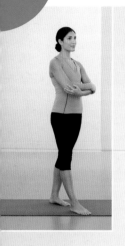

21 Roll up to standing and place one foot ahead of the other, about your foot's distance and a hand-width apart. Hold onto something if you cannot keep your balance, otherwise fold your arms in front of you and hold onto your elbows. Firm the hips and pull your navel to your spine (see p.19). Inhale, then tuck your chin under and round your upper back, allowing your head to hang.

22 Exhale, scoop deeper into your spine, and lower your head to hip-height as if you were going over an imaginary fence. Repeat 2 more times, then change legs and repeat on the other side.

take the feet a hand-width apart

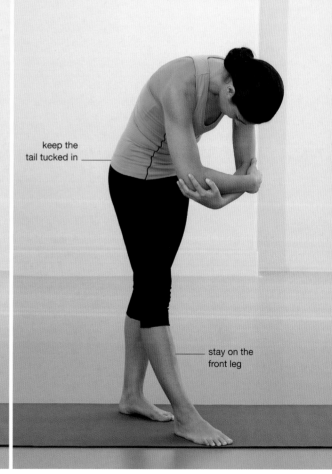

keep the tail tucked in

stay on the front leg

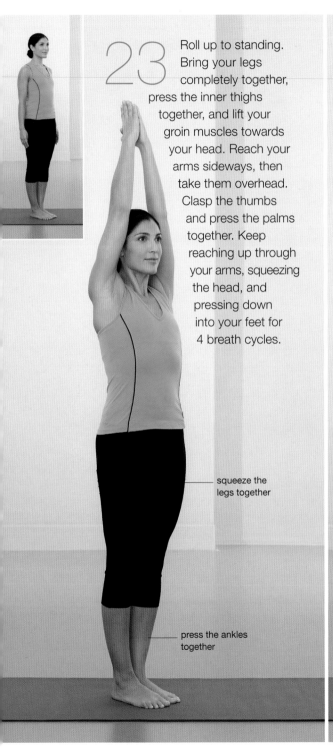

23 Roll up to standing. Bring your legs completely together, press the inner thighs together, and lift your groin muscles towards your head. Reach your arms sideways, then take them overhead. Clasp the thumbs and press the palms together. Keep reaching up through your arms, squeezing the head, and pressing down into your feet for 4 breath cycles.

squeeze the legs together

press the ankles together

24 Lower your arms and shake them gently to release the tension. Repeat, then gently move your body to release any tension.

posture stretch at a glance

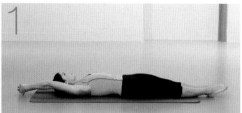

▲ Elongations, p.42

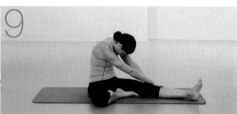

▲ Elongations, p.42

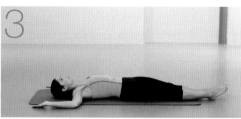

▲ "W's", p.43

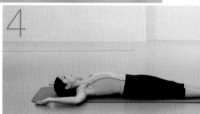

▲ "W's", p.43

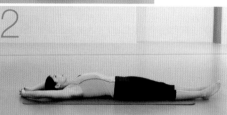

▲ Hurdler lat stretch, p.46

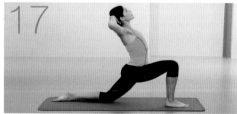

▲ Hurdler lat stretch, p.46

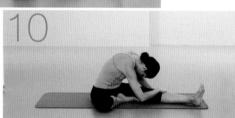

▲ Balance point stretch, p.47

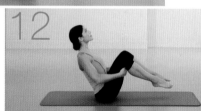

▲ Balance point stretch, p.47

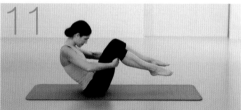

▲ Lunge opener p.50

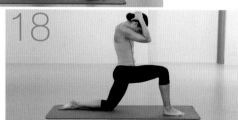

▲ Lunge opener, p.50

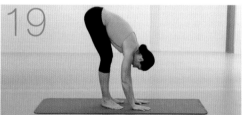

▲ Round back squat, p.51

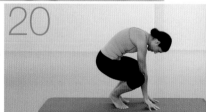

▲ Round back squat, p.51

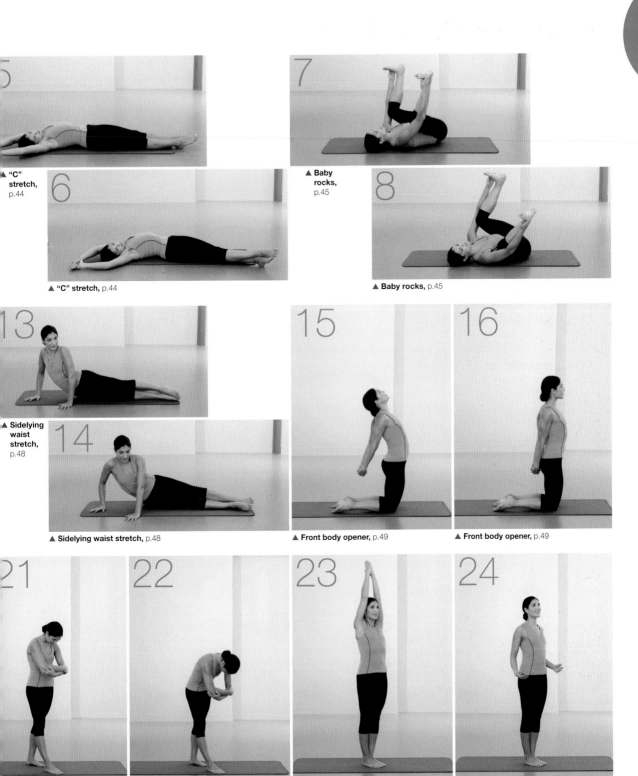

▲ "C" stretch, p.44

▲ "C" stretch, p.44

▲ Baby rocks, p.45

▲ Baby rocks, p.45

▲ Sidelying waist stretch, p.48

▲ Sidelying waist stretch, p.48

▲ Front body opener, p.49

▲ Front body opener, p.49

▲ Hanging stretch, p.52

▲ Hanging stretch, p.52

▲ Top-to-toe stretch, p.53

▲ Top-to-toe stretch, p.53

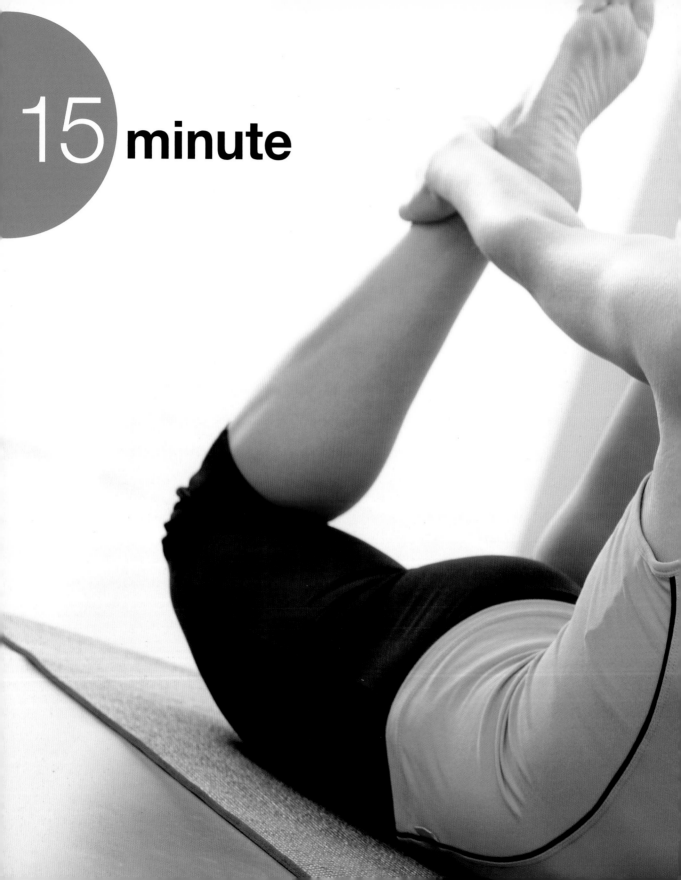

15 minute

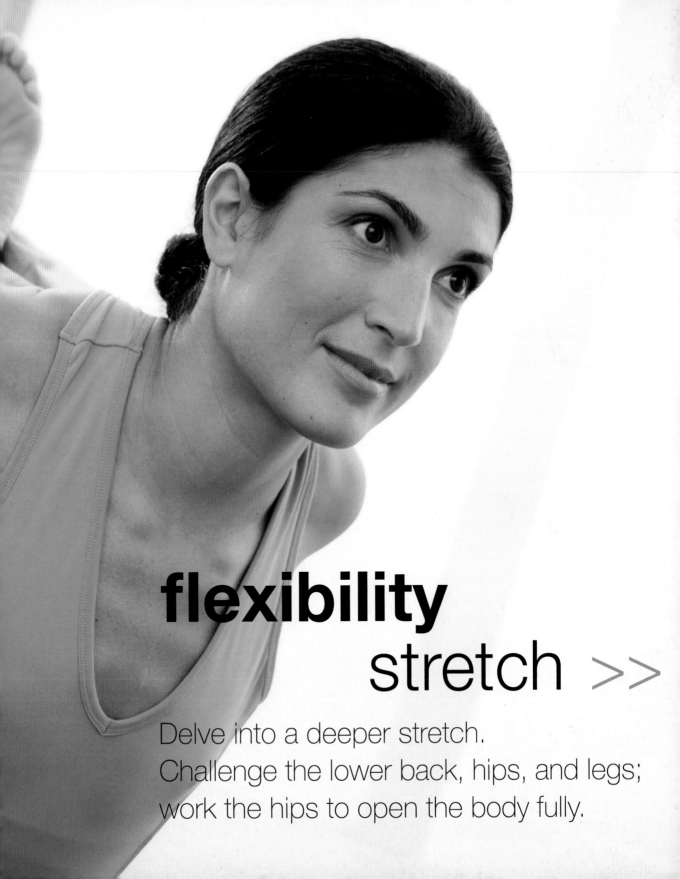

flexibility
stretch >>

Delve into a deeper stretch.
Challenge the lower back, hips, and legs;
work the hips to open the body fully.

>> **flexibility** stretch

Flexibility is best understood as developing your own potential. Each body is unique, with its own set of bone shapes and muscle lengths. Take the challenge here to continue opening your entire body through the gateway of the hips. Hip suppleness is essential to spinal health.

The best way to achieve full body flexibility is to take on the challenge of the lower back, hips, and legs. Many people give up when they feel they are not flexible in the hamstrings, but remember that the body also comprises fascial tissue (see p.12) that, amongst other roles, ties the biomechanics of the upper body to that of the lower body. Now that you've done some loosening and lengthening of your whole body, it's time to focus on a deeper opening of your lower body. This sequence offers more moves that combine stretches with circular, rotational movements. It may require more modification than the first two workouts. Take heart. Challenging yourself with many different exercises will help you to identify your weak areas. There is always a back door into a movement – a way in which you can break the movement down and simply perform parts of it until they transform into old, familiar friends. Then you can join them together again and you're there!

The exercises

The Knee pumps prepare the legs and hips for the next moves. Part of my daily ritual, Knee pumps help to keep my knees and sciatic nerves – the long nerve along the backs of the legs – supple. There is no harm, and it is very beneficial, if you take the extra time to increase the repetitions to as many as 20 on each leg.

The Quad stretch, Thigh sweep, Fouetté stretch, and Figure 4 stretch are absolutely essential to my personal regime. Go slowly at first and take

> >> **tips for** flexibility stretch
>
> - **Suspend judgement** about your hip and leg stretch. Slow, steady persistence pays off. Look to yourself, and in yourself, for comparison.
>
> - **Be sure to energize** your upper body as well as your lower body to create the necessary full-body connection.
>
> - **Always use straps**, belts, or bands to modify when needed.
>
> - **Changing the length of tight**, stiff muscles takes time. If your body type is over-flexible, tighten yourself and make the motion or position smaller so as not to over-stretch.

care to observe the transitions from one movement to the next. Work hard to make these transitions smooth; they are actually additional stretches that help to give the sequence its three-dimensional element.

Challenge yourself to master the sequence by imagining you are coaching someone and have to demonstrate and explain each move to them. Being a teacher forces you to think about the nature of each movement and is the best way to clarify the movements in your own mind.

When you get to Lying hamstring stretch and Advancing frogs, work hard to coordinate all the various parts. It may seem overwhelming to think of them all at once, so first start with the obvious – the basic shape. Again, modify, modify, modify. Rome wasn't built in a day. The next two moves, the Straddle and the Pull-the-thread lunge give you a bit of a rest.

Do try the Angel flight stretch. Remember, your shape and range will be different to our beautiful model's, so start low and slow. This stretch is the ultimate in opening the entire front of the pelvis and thighs. Stick with it, and I promise you will be transformed beyond all your expectations.

The Cobbler stretch is the gateway to opening the stretch of the hips. In this position, it is important to respect the "voice" of the knees and not over-stretch.

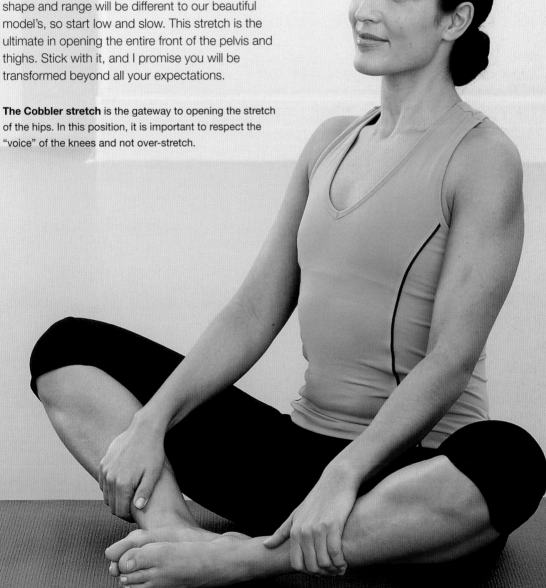

>> knee pumps

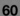

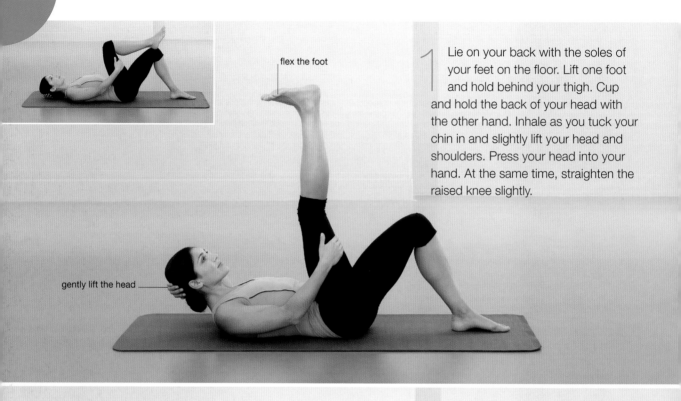

flex the foot

gently lift the head

1 Lie on your back with the soles of your feet on the floor. Lift one foot and hold behind your thigh. Cup and hold the back of your head with the other hand. Inhale as you tuck your chin in and slightly lift your head and shoulders. Press your head into your hand. At the same time, straighten the raised knee slightly.

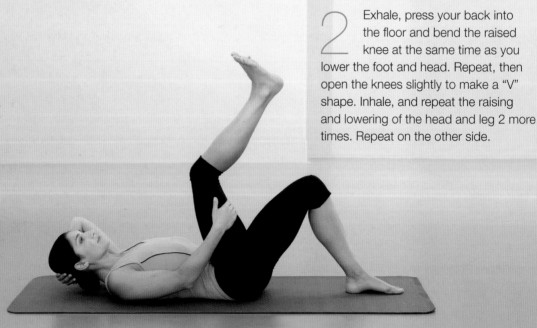

2 Exhale, press your back into the floor and bend the raised knee at the same time as you lower the foot and head. Repeat, then open the knees slightly to make a "V" shape. Inhale, and repeat the raising and lowering of the head and leg 2 more times. Repeat on the other side.

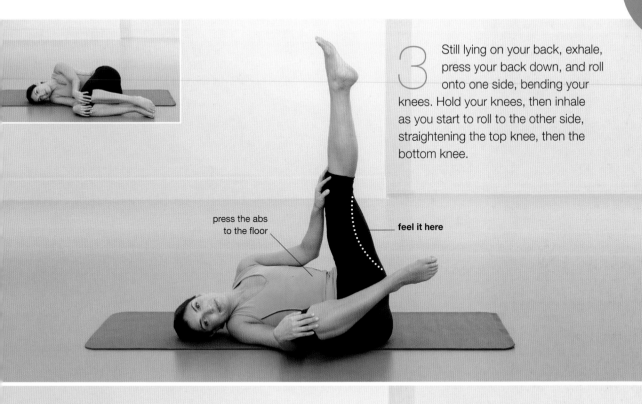

3 Still lying on your back, exhale, press your back down, and roll onto one side, bending your knees. Hold your knees, then inhale as you start to roll to the other side, straightening the top knee, then the bottom knee.

press the abs to the floor

feel it here

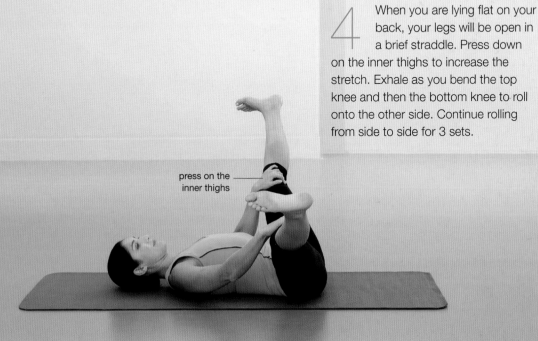

4 When you are lying flat on your back, your legs will be open in a brief straddle. Press down on the inner thighs to increase the stretch. Exhale as you bend the top knee and then the bottom knee to roll onto the other side. Continue rolling from side to side for 3 sets.

press on the inner thighs

>> **cobbler stretch**

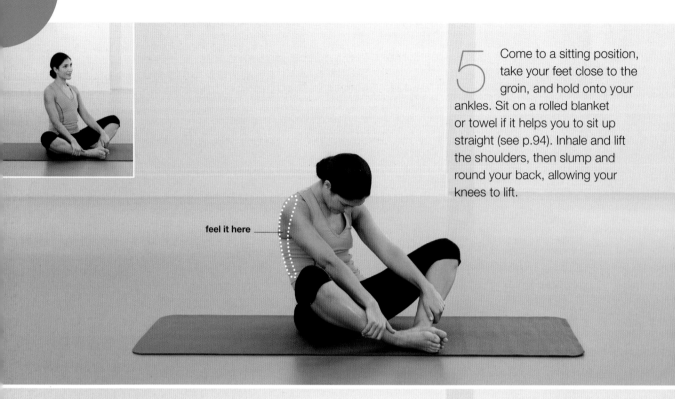

5 Come to a sitting position, take your feet close to the groin, and hold onto your ankles. Sit on a rolled blanket or towel if it helps you to sit up straight (see p.94). Inhale and lift the shoulders, then slump and round your back, allowing your knees to lift.

feel it here ____

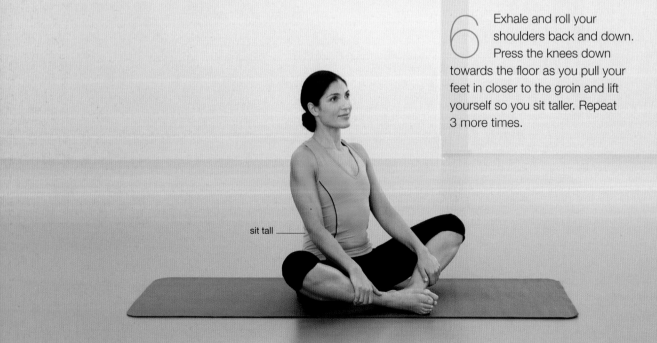

6 Exhale and roll your shoulders back and down. Press the knees down towards the floor as you pull your feet in closer to the groin and lift yourself so you sit taller. Repeat 3 more times.

sit tall ____

>> **quad stretch**

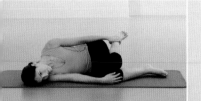

7 Lie on your side and bend both knees up towards your chest. Hold onto your bottom knee. Use a pillow under your neck if you feel any strain (see p.94). Inhale, hold onto your top ankle and pull your top knee gently towards your chest.

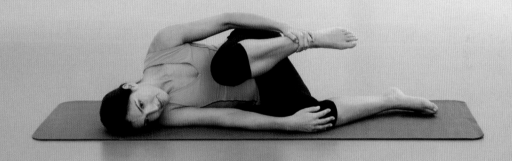

8 Exhale, then smoothly pull your top knee back. Do not let the bottom knee be pulled backwards by the top leg. Stay, then pull backwards a little more on the top knee. Repeat. Release your ankle and go onto your back, then return to your side and straighten your legs.

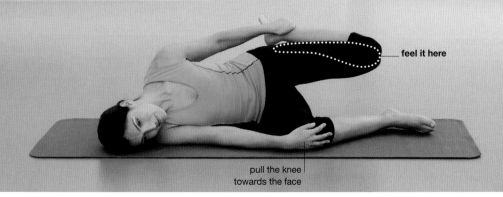

feel it here

pull the knee towards the face

>> thigh sweep

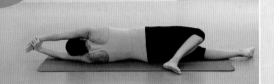

9 Take your arms overhead on the floor and bend your top knee backwards. Hold the wrist on the side of the bent leg, then inhale and slowly pull your wrist out and beyond your head as you roll backwards towards the floor. Do not force it, and modify the position of the knee if you find it uncomfortable.

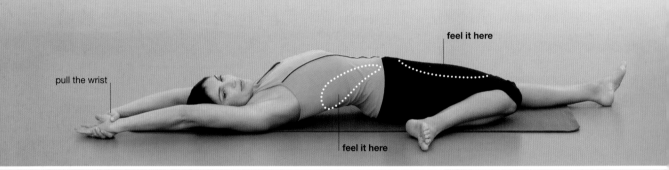

feel it here

pull the wrist

feel it here

10 Exhale, tuck your pelvis under, pull your wrist again, and roll to face forward towards the floor. Repeat, inhaling as you roll backwards and exhaling as you roll forward.

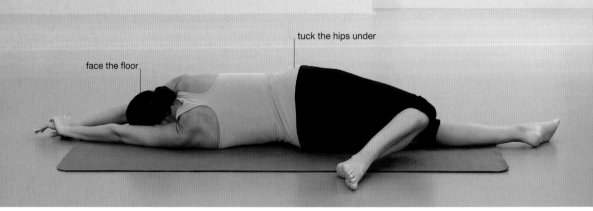

tuck the hips under

face the floor

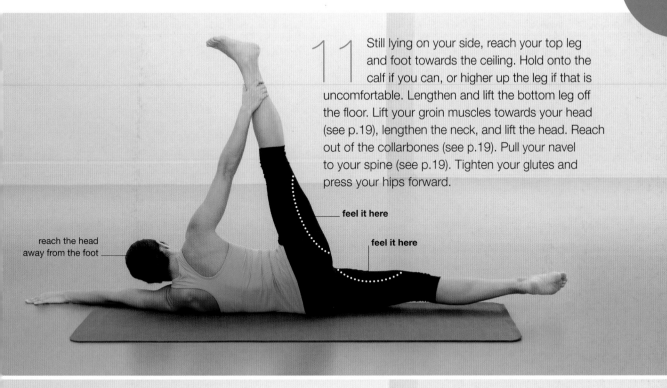

11 Still lying on your side, reach your top leg and foot towards the ceiling. Hold onto the calf if you can, or higher up the leg if that is uncomfortable. Lengthen and lift the bottom leg off the floor. Lift your groin muscles towards your head (see p.19), lengthen the neck, and lift the head. Reach out of the collarbones (see p.19). Pull your navel to your spine (see p.19). Tighten your glutes and press your hips forward.

feel it here

feel it here

reach the head away from the foot

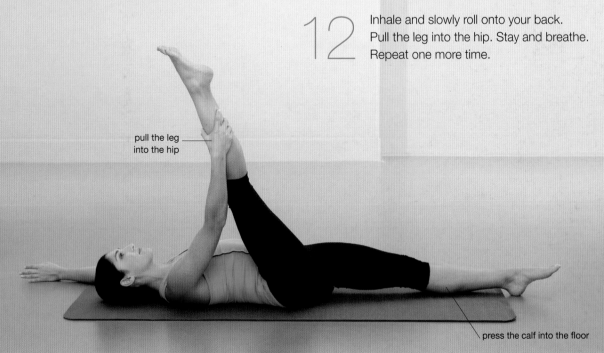

12 Inhale and slowly roll onto your back. Pull the leg into the hip. Stay and breathe. Repeat one more time.

pull the leg into the hip

press the calf into the floor

>> **figure 4 stretch**

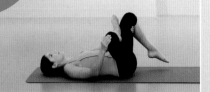

13 Go onto your back, bend your knees, and place one ankle on the other thigh. Place one hand underneath that thigh and the palm of the other hand on the knee of the crossed leg. Lift the groin muscles towards the head to stabilize the spine. Inhale and pull the hand behind the thigh towards your chest.

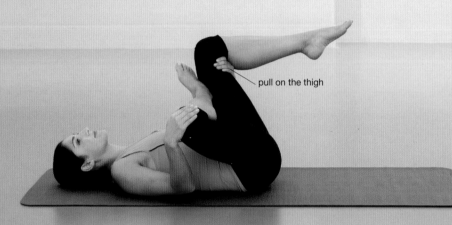

pull on the thigh

14 Exhale and press the hand against the knee, away from your face, keeping the bent leg parallel to the floor. If the knee hurts, come out of the position, or loosen the posture. Repeat. Release both legs, thump your thighs, and breathe normally. Roll onto the other side and repeat Steps 7 to 14.

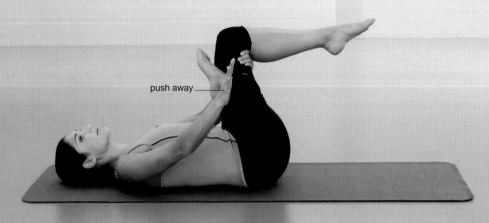

push away

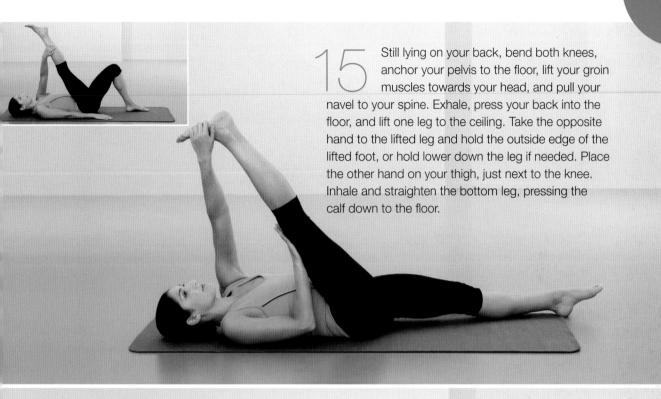

15 Still lying on your back, bend both knees, anchor your pelvis to the floor, lift your groin muscles towards your head, and pull your navel to your spine. Exhale, press your back into the floor, and lift one leg to the ceiling. Take the opposite hand to the lifted leg and hold the outside edge of the lifted foot, or hold lower down the leg if needed. Place the other hand on your thigh, just next to the knee. Inhale and straighten the bottom leg, pressing the calf down to the floor.

16 Exhale and lift the head. Gently press the hand on the thigh away from you. The top foot pulls your leg into the hip socket. Stay for 2 breath cycles, then repeat on the other side. Gently release the legs and thump your thighs against the floor.

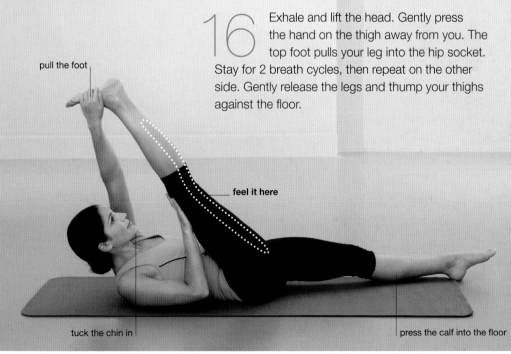

pull the foot

feel it here

tuck the chin in

press the calf into the floor

>> **advancing frogs**

17 Come onto your hands and knees, open your knees, reach your arms forward, and squat back, bringing your hips close to your heels. Support your back by lifting the abs. Stay for 2 breath cycles.

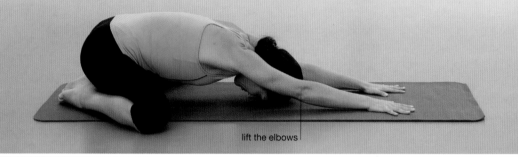

lift the elbows

18 Move your torso and arms forward, and come up on your forearms. Actively press the inner edges of your heels into the floor. Your heels will come apart. Lift the groin muscles towards the head to avoid slumping in the lower back. Stay for 2 breath cycles.

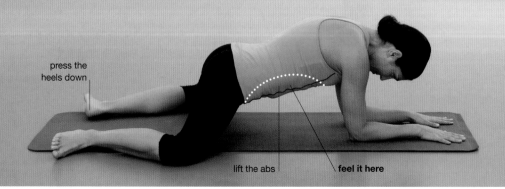

press the heels down

lift the abs

feel it here

19 Come to a sitting position, sitting evenly on your sitting bones, with your legs open to at least a 90° angle, and with your toes pulled towards your head. Lift your back and open your chest. Sit on a rolled blanket or towel if it helps you to sit up straight, or bend your knees. Lift the groin muscles up towards the head. Open your arms strongly sideways and reach out through the head, legs, and arms.

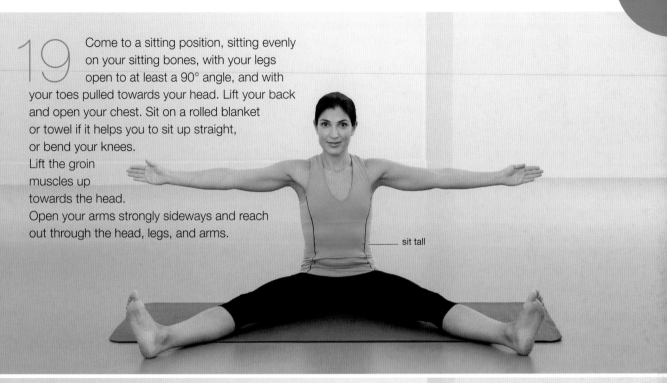

sit tall

20 Inhale and reach up and over an imaginary fence to one side. Rest the lower hand on the floor behind the outstretched leg. Firm your waist. Exhale, then return to centre by "painting the ceiling" with your top arm. Repeat on the other side, then release. Gently roll your shoulders to relax.

reach through the third finger

pull the navel to the spine

lean on the back hand

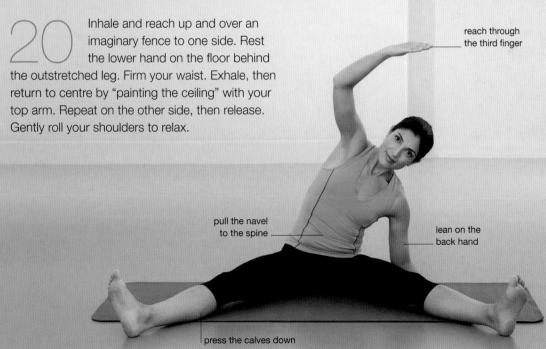

press the calves down

>> pull-the-thread lunge

21 Go onto your hands and knees, take one leg in front, and lean into it, palms either side of the front foot. Line up the bent-leg knee and toes straight ahead in front of the hip. Press the foot into the floor. Extend the other leg straight behind you and tuck the pelvis under strongly.

tuck the tail under

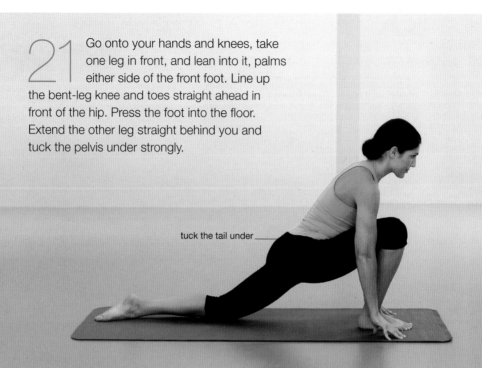

22 Pull an imaginary thread up to the ceiling with the hand on the side of the extended leg. Look up at the hand and press down into the floor with your other hand. Stay for 2 breath cycles. Take the hand down to the floor, then repeat with the other leg in front.

look at the "thread"

tighten the waist

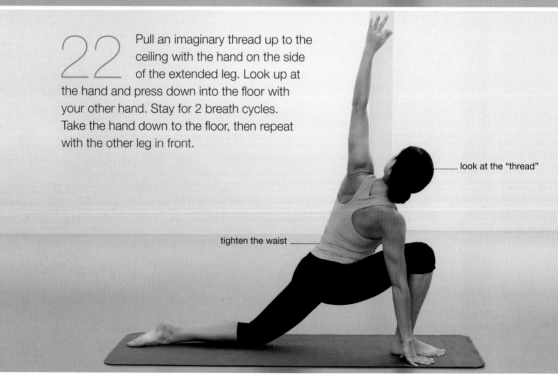

>> flexibility stretch

>> **angel flight stretch**

23 Lie on your stomach, face turned to one side. Feel the imaginary swimming-pool water lifting your abdomen off the floor (see p.18). Press the tailbone down towards the heels. Inhale, then reach back and bend the knees to hold onto your ankles.

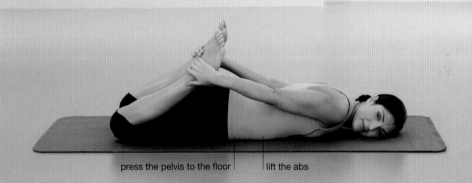

press the pelvis to the floor | lift the abs

24 Exhale, press your feet against your hands, and lift your chest and thighs off the floor to make a bow-like shape. Stay for 2 breath cycles, then release your hands and feet and relax for another 2 breath cycles, breathing deeply.

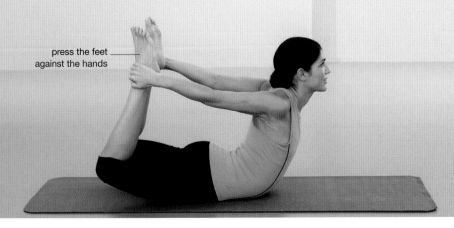

press the feet
against the hands

flexibility stretch at a glance

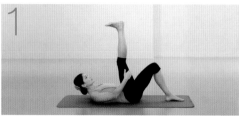

▲ Knee pumps, p.60

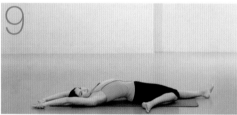

▲ Knee pumps, p.60

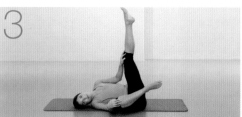

▲ Baby rolls, p.61

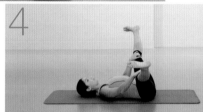

▲ Baby rolls, p.61

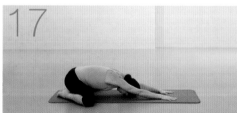

▲ Thigh sweep, p.64

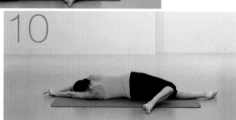

▲ Thigh sweep, p.64

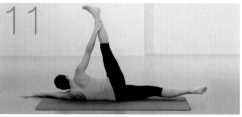

▲ Fouetté stretch, p.65

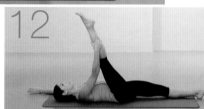

▲ Fouetté stretch, p.65

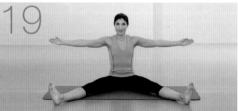

▲ Advancing frogs, p.68

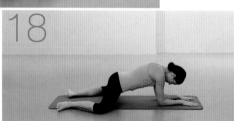

▲ Advancing frogs, p.68

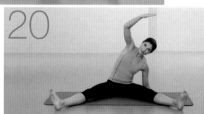

▲ Straddle, p.69

▲ Straddle, p.69

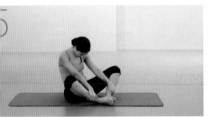

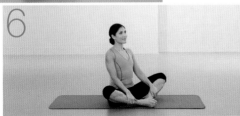

Cobbler stretch, p.62

▲ Cobbler stretch, p.62

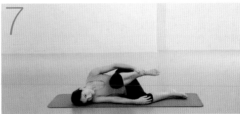

▲ **Quad stretch,** p.63

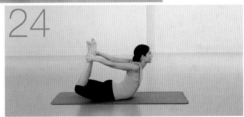

▲ Quad stretch, p.63

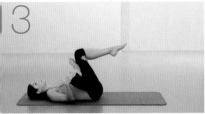

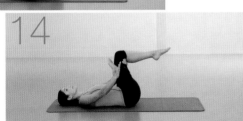

Figure 4 stretch, p.66

▲ Figure 4 stretch, p.66

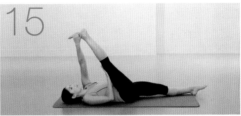

▲ **Lying hamstring stretch,** p.67

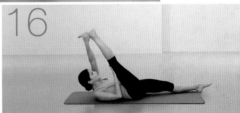

▲ Lying hamstring stretch, p.67

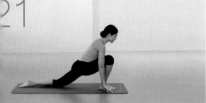

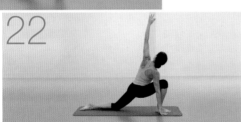

Pull-the-thread lunge, p.70

▲ Pull-the-thread lunge, p.70

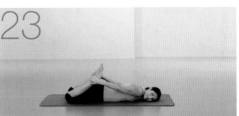

▲ **Angel flight stretch,** p.71

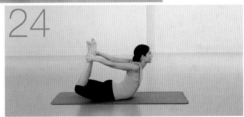

▲ Angel flight stretch, p.71

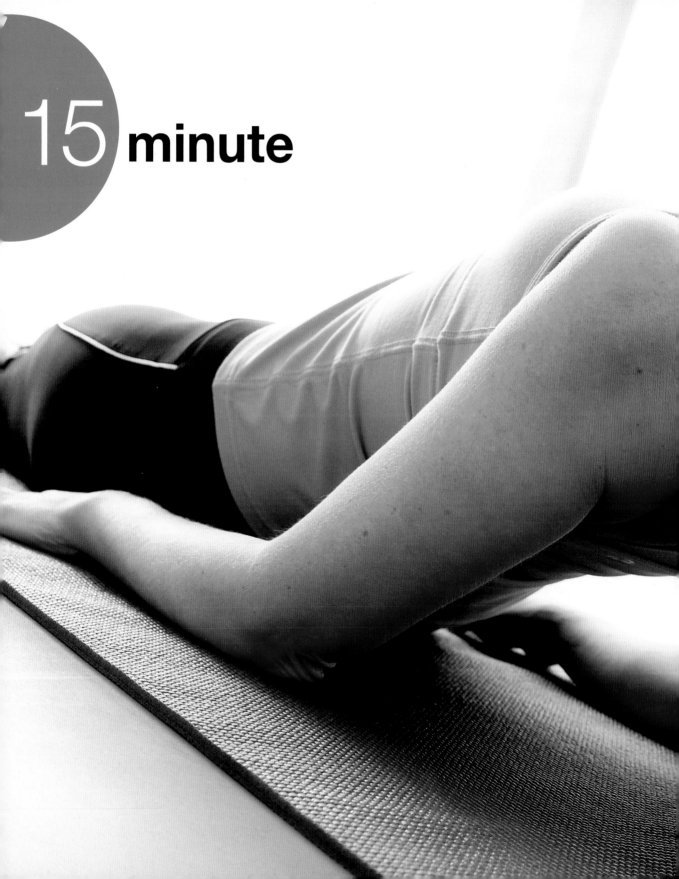

15 minute

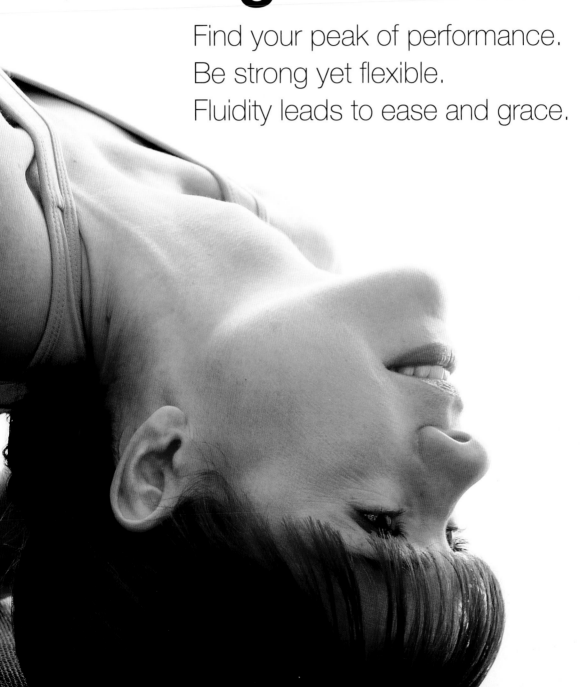

strength stretch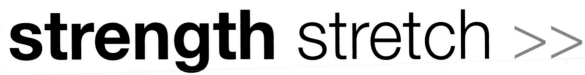

Find your peak of performance.
Be strong yet flexible.
Fluidity leads to ease and grace.

>> **strength** stretch

You don't need to be a contortionist to master this final sequence. Use your body control to guide you into these more advanced movements. Regard it as your ultimate goal. Even beginners can discover how much control they need to exert, whether they are trying to balance in a precarious pose or performing the simplest stretch.

Strength by definition means grounding and control. See this sequence as one feat of strength after another in an Olympic trial. Close up, you can see the suppleness of an athlete's body, and in action you can see the litheness of their motions. Think of all the hours of preparation Olympic athletes must endure to reach their final goal. In this sequence, look at each exercise as a goal in and of itself. The trick is to break each exercise down by starting small and gradually building to a larger and steadier range of motion. Remember that achieving a general level of fitness takes about two months of practice, and developing a split may take more like six months, depending on how naturally flexible you are. The recipe for Olympic development is to stress the body, then to rest it. Be wise and give your body a good rest after practising this sequence. The poses and movements here move towards a crescendo that primes you for success.

The exercises
Set the tone for strength by standing tall in the Butterfly stretch and the Upper side bend. Feel your upper body moving against the lower body, as if your lower body were rooted and anchored, like a great oak tree. The series of squats that follows coordinates the strength and suppleness of the spine with the suppleness of the legs. Get more benefit by opening your knees as wide as you can in the Wide squat twist and in the

> ## >> **tips for** strength stretch
>
> - **Think of your spine** and legs grounded like the trunk and roots of a great oak tree.
> - **Remember, you're not failing** if you need to use props and smaller positions to help you get familiar with the exercises.
> - **Find your "pelvic diaphragm"**, and keep looking for ways to coordinate your inner muscle strength as you work with larger movements.
> - **Always be careful** with large stretches of the neck. Never pull on the head.

Deep squat. These squats also provide a great opportunity to strengthen the "pelvic diaphragm" – the parachute-like muscle layer that lies at the bottom of the torso.

As you perform the next exercise, the Neck stretch, bear in mind that you are now coordinating the "neck diaphragm" – the parachute-like muscle and soft tissue layers defining the top of the rib cage – with the pelvic diaphragm. So this sequence works on more levels than meet the eye. It is the ultimate in strength and control. Become willing to acquire the ability to coordinate deep muscles with the larger, more obvious muscles, such as the abs, the glutes, and the thighs.

Continue this coordination as you now ripple the spine more strongly in the Kneeling cat and the Kneeling side stretch. The goal is not whether you can approximate the position, but whether you can take such a rangy pose and still coordinate the deeper muscles. Keep this concept activated in the Fish stretch. The last three exercises are the most challenging of all. Have faith in yourself, and know that little steps make big leaps possible. Modify. Go slowly. Every attempt warrants a gold star. Keep your eyes on the prize, which is the combination of stretch with control. Fulfil the potential of your body, one step at a time.

Connecting the deeper core muscles while tensing the larger, outer muscles in these strength stretches adds value and effectiveness to your work.

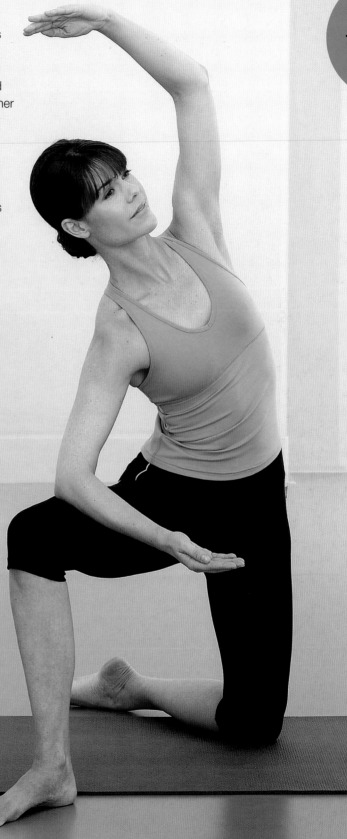

>> **butterfly stretch**

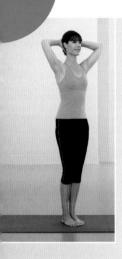

1 Stand with legs completely together and pressing the base of the big and little toes, and the middle of the heel of both feet on the floor. Lift your groin muscles towards the head (see p.19). Pull your navel to your spine (see p.19). Clasp your hands behind your head, inhale, and lift up and forward from your waist. Simultaneously bow your head, bend your knees, and bring the elbows towards each other.

2 Exhale, straighten the legs, and stretch up and out of your waist, fanning the elbows open. Reach out through the points of the elbows and feel as if your breastbone is being pulled up towards the ceiling. Repeat, then relax and shake the hands.

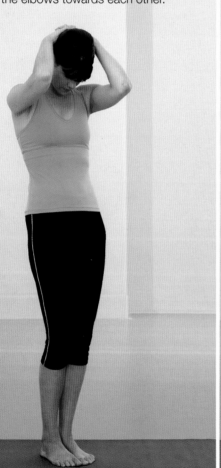

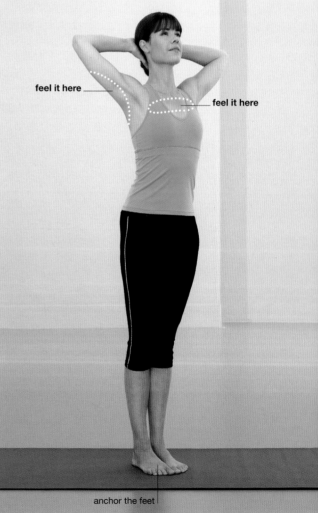

feel it here

feel it here

anchor the feet

3 Still with your legs completely together, renew your form. Lift the groin muscles towards the head, and pull the abs up and into your spine. Clasp your hands behind your head.

4 Inhale and lift up and out of the rib cage, over an imaginary fence under one armpit. Tilt one elbow down towards the floor, the other up towards the ceiling. Exhale and take your shoulders back to centre. Feel a "V" of strength from the small of the lower back to the points of the elbows. Repeat on the other side, and then repeat one more set.

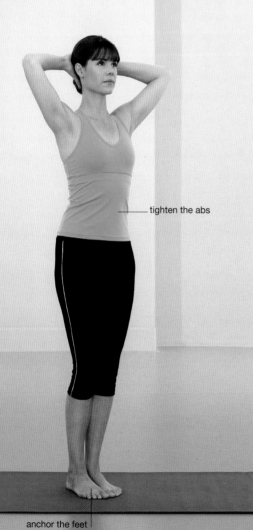

tighten the abs

anchor the feet

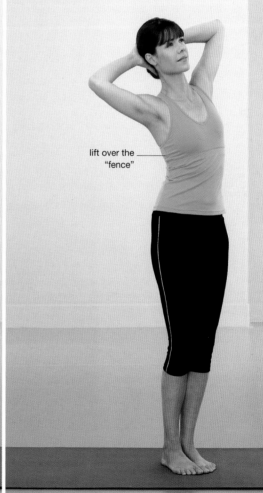

lift over the "fence"

>> **flat back squat**

5 Lift the abs and roll down your spine into a squatting position. Let your knees open and go onto the balls of your feet. Lean on your hands, then inhale as you lift diagonally up and out with your chest, keeping your back flat and extended. Imagine you are looking under a table.

6 Exhale slowly as you lift the hips upwards, taking the heels as high as you can. Straighten your knees and tuck your chin into the legs. Keep lifting the groin muscles towards the head. Stay and breathe, then repeat, intensifying the stretch at the end. Lower and relax. Repeat.

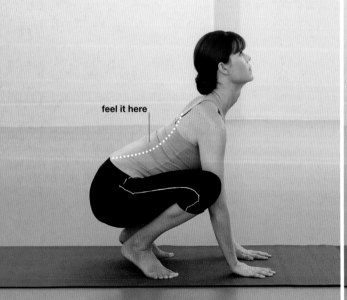

feel it here

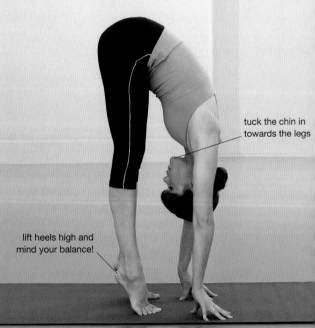

tuck the chin in towards the legs

lift heels high and mind your balance!

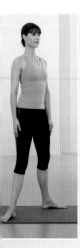

7 Come to a standing position with your feet wider than hip-width apart and your toes facing outwards. Lift the groin muscles towards the head, inhale, and lower your hips. Bring your hands to the thighs, take some of your weight into them, and check that your toes are in line with your knees.

8 Inhale, press backwards on one hand on the inside of the knee, twisting that shoulder down. Look up and out in the opposite direction. Stay for 2 breath cycles, then exhale and bring the shoulders back to centre. Come up, shake your legs a little, and repeat on the other side.

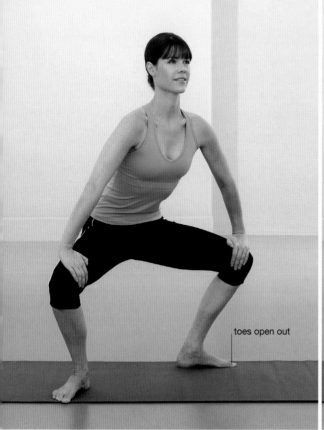

toes open out

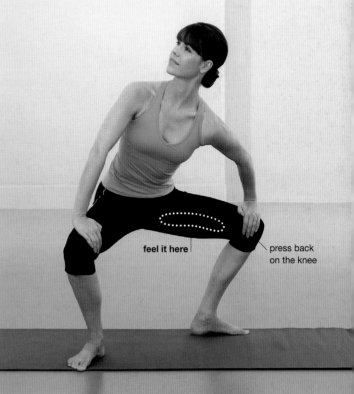

feel it here

press back on the knee

>> **deep squat**

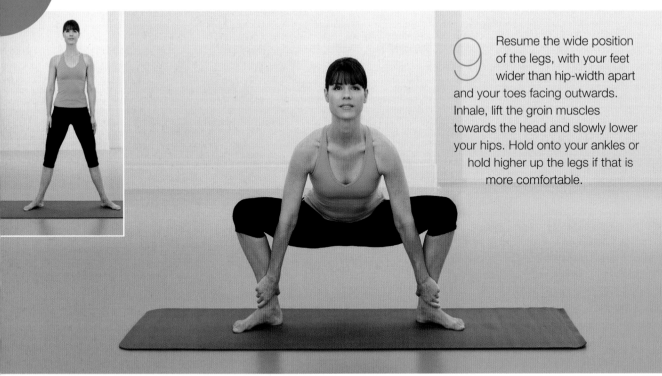

9 Resume the wide position of the legs, with your feet wider than hip-width apart and your toes facing outwards. Inhale, lift the groin muscles towards the head and slowly lower your hips. Hold onto your ankles or hold higher up the legs if that is more comfortable.

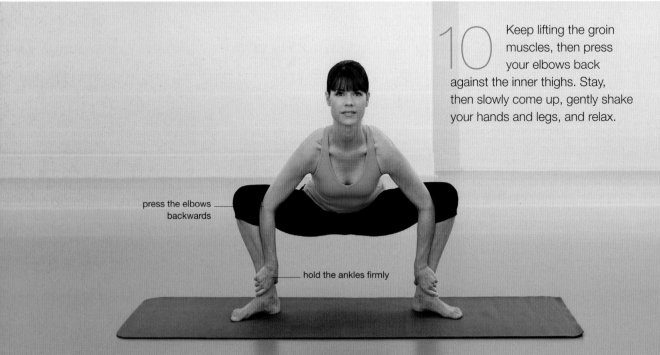

10 Keep lifting the groin muscles, then press your elbows back against the inner thighs. Stay, then slowly come up, gently shake your hands and legs, and relax.

press the elbows backwards

hold the ankles firmly

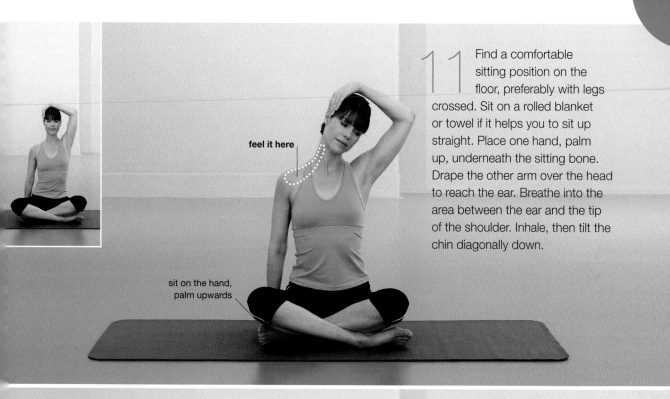

feel it here

sit on the hand, palm upwards

11 Find a comfortable sitting position on the floor, preferably with legs crossed. Sit on a rolled blanket or towel if it helps you to sit up straight. Place one hand, palm up, underneath the sitting bone. Drape the other arm over the head to reach the ear. Breathe into the area between the ear and the tip of the shoulder. Inhale, then tilt the chin diagonally down.

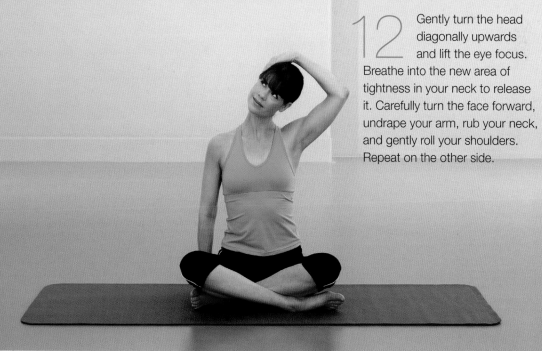

12 Gently turn the head diagonally upwards and lift the eye focus. Breathe into the new area of tightness in your neck to release it. Carefully turn the face forward, undrape your arm, rub your neck, and gently roll your shoulders. Repeat on the other side.

>> **kneeling cat**

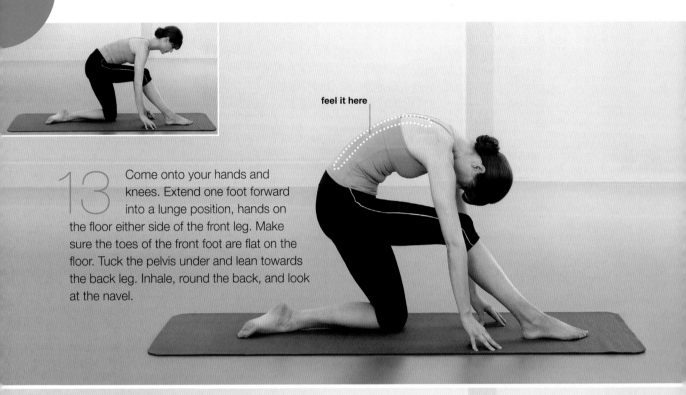

feel it here

13 Come onto your hands and knees. Extend one foot forward into a lunge position, hands on the floor either side of the front leg. Make sure the toes of the front foot are flat on the floor. Tuck the pelvis under and lean towards the back leg. Inhale, round the back, and look at the navel.

14 Open your mouth, exhale from the back of the throat, lengthen your lower back, then start arching your back and lifting your chest. Imagine you are looking under a table. Repeat, inhaling and rounding, and exhaling and arching. Repeat on the other side.

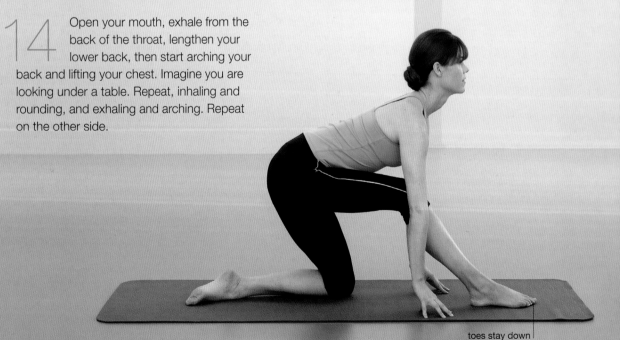

toes stay down

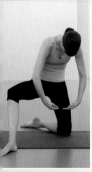

15 Starting on your hands and knees, take one leg diagonally in front, knee bent, sole of the foot on the floor. Turn both legs out slightly, lower the head, and take the arms in front of you, touching your third fingers together. Then roll up through the spine and fan your arms open sideways.

16 Tuck your pelvis under and reach your top arm up and over towards the bent leg. Rest your lower forearm on the thigh of the bent leg. Reach up and out through the third finger of the top arm. Lift the groin muscles towards the head. Stay for 3 breath cycles, then repeat on the other side.

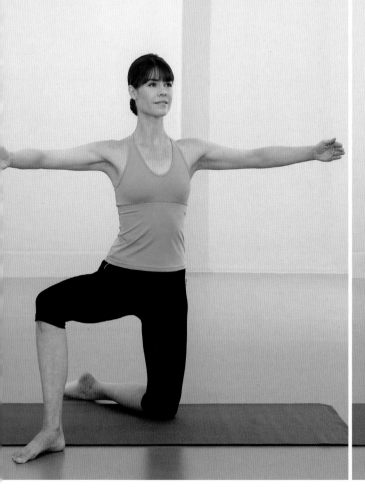

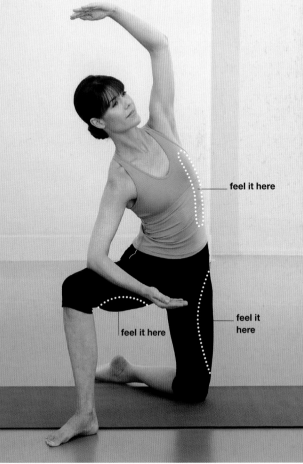

feel it here

feel it here

feel it here

>> **fish stretch**

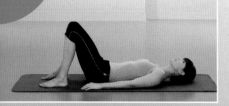

17 Lie on your back, knees bent, soles of the feet on the floor. Place your palms on the floor by your hips. Exhale, then gently press the lower back forward and arch your back slightly.

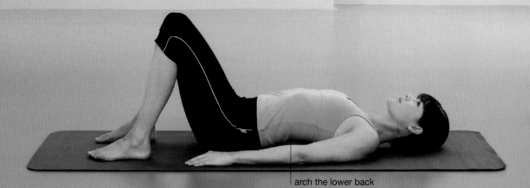

arch the lower back

18 Roll your shoulder blades back and down, then press down on your forearms, and arch your back more to come up onto the top of your head. Put as little pressure on the head as possible. Stay for 1 long breath cycle. Relax, then repeat.

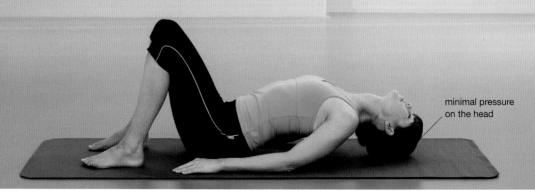

minimal pressure on the head

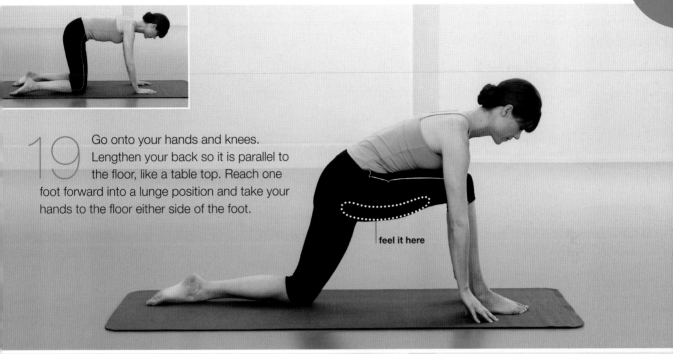

19 Go onto your hands and knees. Lengthen your back so it is parallel to the floor, like a table top. Reach one foot forward into a lunge position and take your hands to the floor either side of the foot.

feel it here

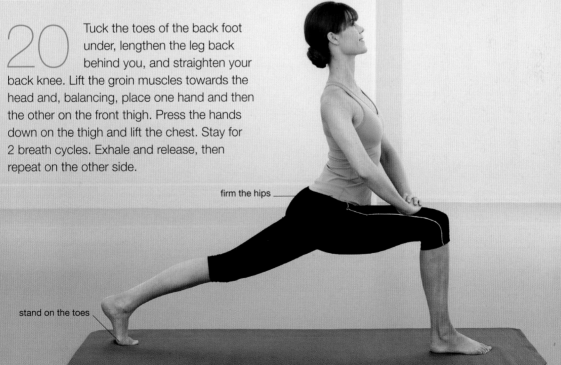

20 Tuck the toes of the back foot under, lengthen the leg back behind you, and straighten your back knee. Lift the groin muscles towards the head and, balancing, place one hand and then the other on the front thigh. Press the hands down on the thigh and lift the chest. Stay for 2 breath cycles. Exhale and release, then repeat on the other side.

firm the hips

stand on the toes

>> **pigeon arabesque**

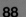

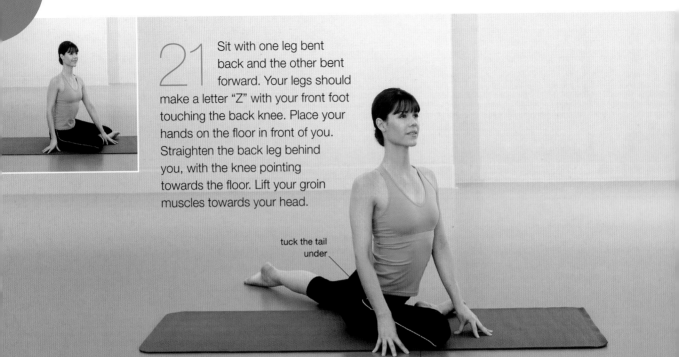

21 Sit with one leg bent back and the other bent forward. Your legs should make a letter "Z" with your front foot touching the back knee. Place your hands on the floor in front of you. Straighten the back leg behind you, with the knee pointing towards the floor. Lift your groin muscles towards your head.

tuck the tail under

balance on the thigh

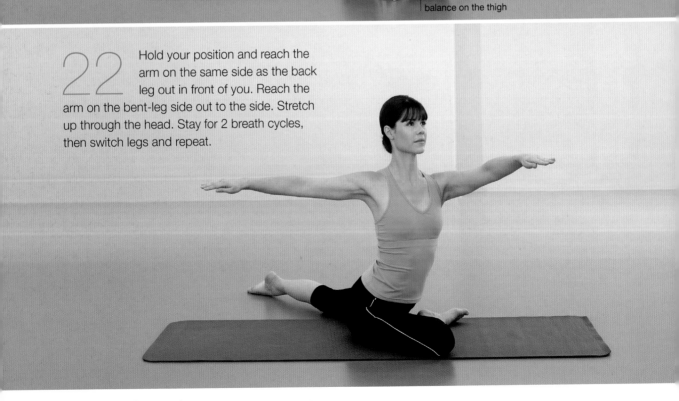

22 Hold your position and reach the arm on the same side as the back leg out in front of you. Reach the arm on the bent-leg side out to the side. Stretch up through the head. Stay for 2 breath cycles, then switch legs and repeat.

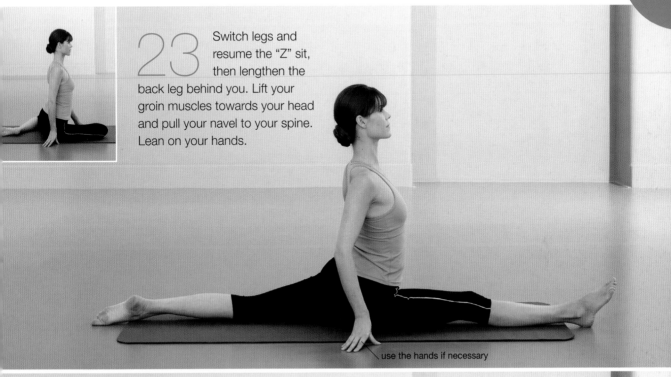

23 Switch legs and resume the "Z" sit, then lengthen the back leg behind you. Lift your groin muscles towards your head and pull your navel to your spine. Lean on your hands.

use the hands if necessary

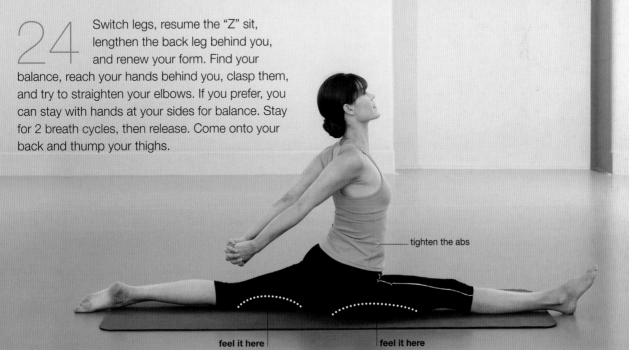

24 Switch legs, resume the "Z" sit, lengthen the back leg behind you, and renew your form. Find your balance, reach your hands behind you, clasp them, and try to straighten your elbows. If you prefer, you can stay with hands at your sides for balance. Stay for 2 breath cycles, then release. Come onto your back and thump your thighs.

tighten the abs

feel it here   feel it here

strength stretch at a glance

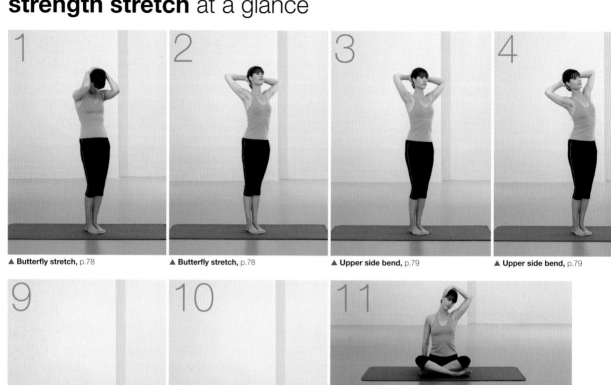

▲ **Butterfly stretch,** p.78

▲ **Butterfly stretch,** p.78

▲ **Upper side bend,** p.79

▲ **Upper side bend,** p.79

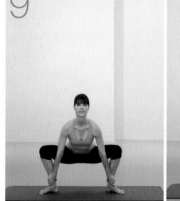

▲ **Deep squat,** p.82

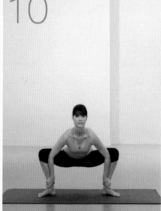

▲ **Deep squat,** p.82

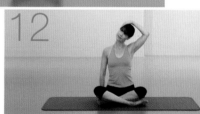

▲ **Neck stretch,** p. 83

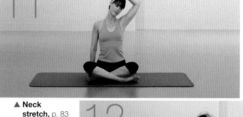

▲ **Neck stretch,** p.83

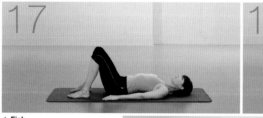

▲ **Fish stretch,** p.86

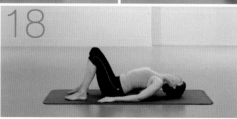

▲ **Fish stretch,** p.86

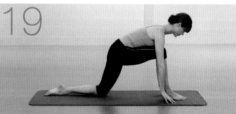

▲ **Thigh lunge,** p.87

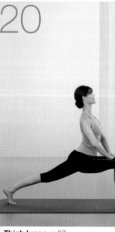

▲ **Thigh lunge,** p.87

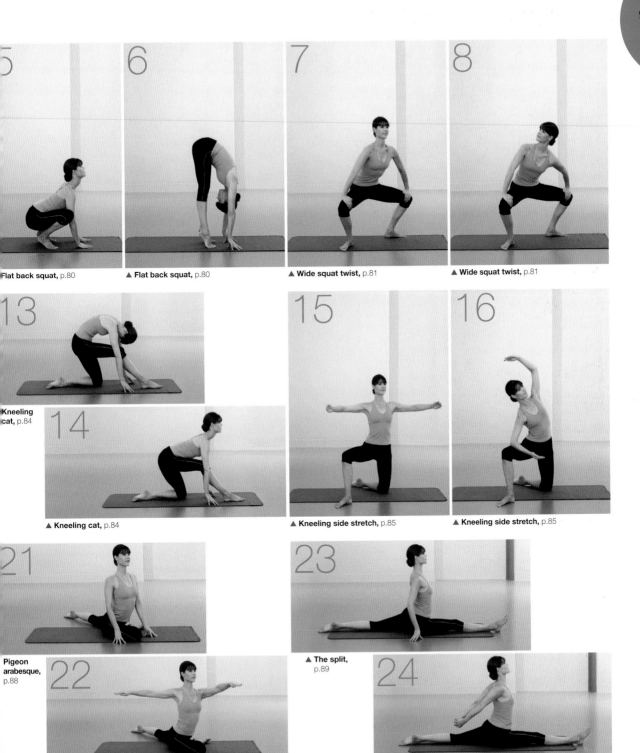

5
6
7
8

Flat back squat, p.80   ▲ Flat back squat, p.80   ▲ Wide squat twist, p.81   ▲ Wide squat twist, p.81

13
14
15
16

Kneeling cat, p.84   ▲ Kneeling cat, p.84   ▲ Kneeling side stretch, p.85   ▲ Kneeling side stretch, p.85

21
22
23
24

Pigeon arabesque, p.88   ▲ Pigeon arabesque, p.88   ▲ The split, p.89   ▲ The split, p.89

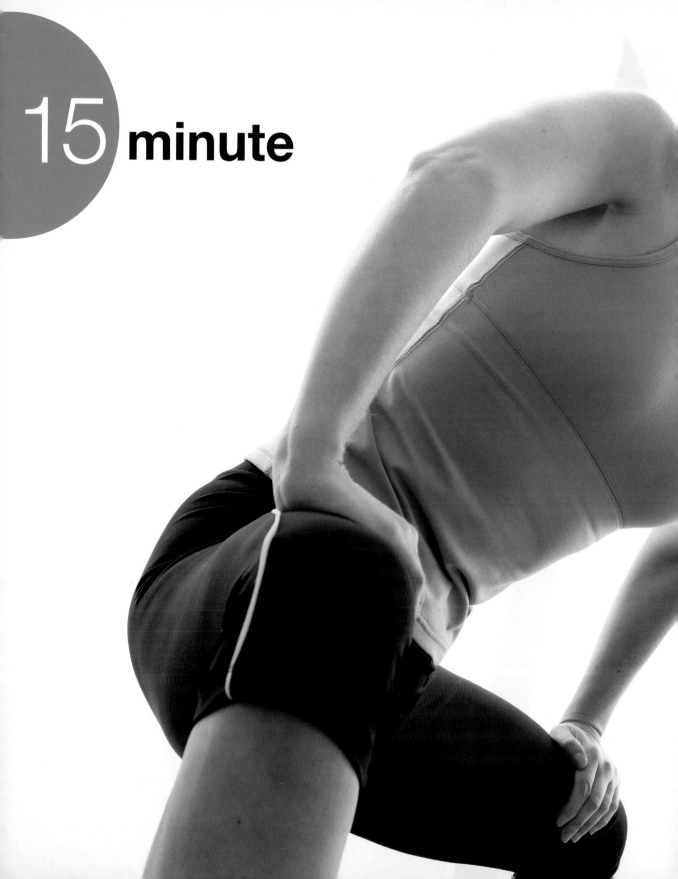

15 minute

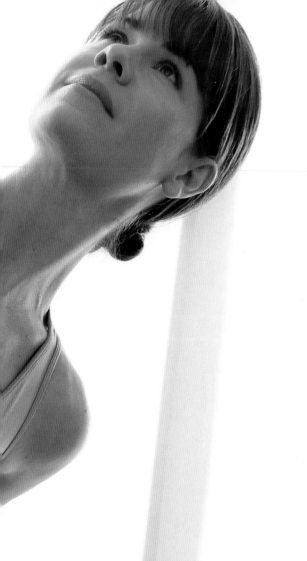

moving on >>

Life propels us into forward
motion and change.
Incorporate stretching to
live a healthy life.

>> **modify** as needed

It's not a failing to change an exercise to suit your needs, whether it's because of pain, age, or stiffness. There's a back door to every stretch. Nor is it cheating to use props and modifications. It's just plain wise.

The body can move in multiple directions with a great deal of ease, yet people are often deterred from doing stretching exercises because they worry about feeling discouraged. We would all love to look like the models featured in this book, but use them to help you see the stretching exercises clearly, not to compare yourself with them.

Some of the stretches may feel a little strange or unusual, especially if you are new to exercise. Part of the reason we stretch in unusual positions is to identify our weak links, so pay attention and focus on what feels too tight, too loose, or painful.

If an exercise doesn't feel right, there's always a way to make it more accessible. Some people have trouble sitting on the floor because they have tight hamstrings, glutes, or tightness in the lower back, or a combination of one or more of these. Sitting on a footstool, ottoman, towel, or bolster can give just the lift needed to make the stretch possible.

Knees should never hurt during stretching. If they feel painful, support them on pillows or bolsters to take the pressure off. Another tip for this pose is to move the feet farther away from the groin.

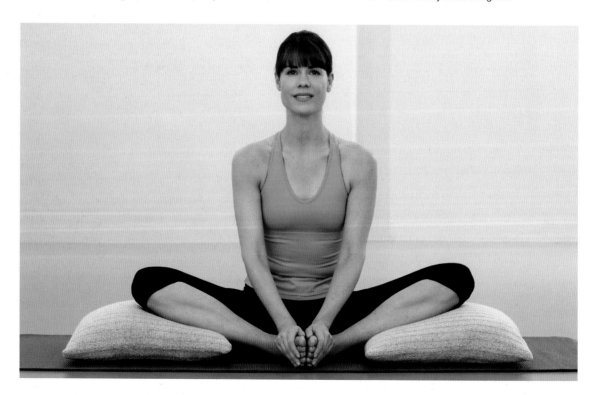

Pay special attention to your knees and monitor them for signs of pain or discomfort. "No pain, no gain" definitely does not apply to these complex joints. If you need to, prop them up with pillows when you are sitting to take the strain off the ligaments. If they feel tender when you kneel on them in weight-bearing positions, support them with some form of padding. Straighten them out of a bent-leg position if it feels uncomfortable. If one of the knees refuses to straighten, as it might in the Lying hamstring stretch (see p.67), use a towel, belt, or strap to reach the foot.

You can increase or decrease the intensity of a stretch as it suits you (perhaps your body feels different on different days or at different times of day) by pulling or extending more or less. Breathing and relaxing help you stretch farther. Alternatively, try modulating the intensity of a stretch by elongating in a progression from one to ten, and then reducing it. The level of intensity should never go into the "strain zone" and you should not have extreme pain after you have performed your stretches. Remember: compare only yourself to yourself to make the greatest gain.

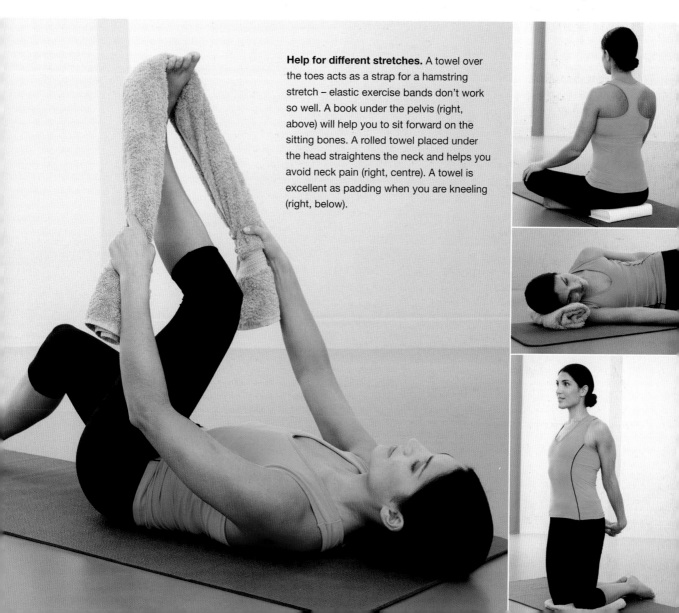

Help for different stretches. A towel over the toes acts as a strap for a hamstring stretch – elastic exercise bands don't work so well. A book under the pelvis (right, above) will help you to sit forward on the sitting bones. A rolled towel placed under the head straightens the neck and helps you avoid neck pain (right, centre). A towel is excellent as padding when you are kneeling (right, below).

>> **stretches for** everyday life

It's easy to take your stretches into everyday life. Notice how you move when you are grooming yourself, dressing, even cooking and cleaning, and turn each movement into a stretch. And think "office" as well as "home" to get the most out of your stretch regime.

Look at the ways your body moves in everyday life. Notice how different movements feel, such as brushing your hair or pulling on a sweater or trousers. Does the task feel comfortable? Do you have the same range of motion on both sides? How does it feel to bend over to reach to a pet? Let your answers to these questions guide you to set yourself goals that will make an action a little easier or smoother.

Gradual changes

Changes to the way we move happen gradually over time. Diminishing range of motion creeps up on people of every age. A student notices writing arm and shoulders tightening during a long exam. A young mother notices a tight chest or sore lower

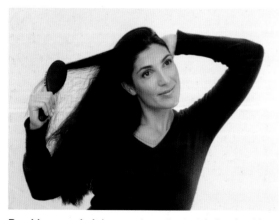

Brushing your hair is a great way to stretch the shoulders and chest. Try switching the brush to your non-dominant hand to balance both sides of the body.

back as she holds or reaches down to a toddler. Older adults notice they can't bend to the floor or reach up into cupboards as easily as before.

Your adaptable body

Life's distractions, such as being preoccupied with a demanding job, with a new baby, or with having to juggle a long commute with household duties can sideline us from regular physical activity. Then suddenly we notice a change and start to worry that our bodies are not as mobile as they once were.

The good news is that your body is adaptable. It changes to accept what the environment is telling it to do. If you inadvertently restrict its movements – for instance, by sitting for long periods – it adapts to the smaller, less frequent motions. Conversely, it can re-adapt. That's why it's important to find ways in everyday life to get an extra little bit of stretch. Small changes can keep your body healthy over time.

In a crowded schedule

It's commendable to devote an hour or two a day to taking exercise, but not everyone can do that. Our 15-minute programmes make it possible to exercise, even with the most crowded schedule. Yet neither should you overlook the power of taking 25 seconds – four breath cycles – to feel the stretch in an everyday position or movement. This will add to your overall physical wellbeing. Using this strategy during those overwhelming times of life, when every second appears to be accountable, will pay rich dividends.

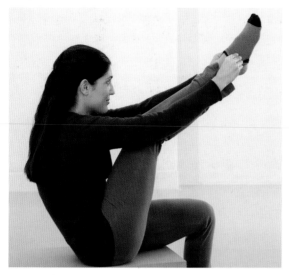

Putting on your socks is a good time for a hamstring stretch. Simply lift the leg, or reach over to it, bow the head, and take a few breaths.

>> **everyday stretches** that
make a difference

- **Reach a little farther** to stretch into that cupboard. Take a break. Yawn to stretch the jaw. Open the eyes and look upwards to open the chest and neck.

- **Stretch your legs and hips** when putting on and taking off clothes. Practise lunges when vacuuming and move your hips from side to side when sweeping.

- **Renew your posture at the office** by squeezing between the shoulder blades and rolling your shoulders. Firm the glutes and sit up tall.

Working in an office gives you a good opportunity to use some chair stretches from the Wake up the stretch programme (see pp.22–35). Reach your hands behind your head and wing your elbows open in a chest stretch. It helps your work day go faster and more smoothly. Sitting work is probably among the most tiring, and it's important to take frequent breaks, even for a few breaths. Office stretches increase clear thinking as well as helping to avoid computer over-use problems that can affect your chest, hands, and arms. Intermittent breathing and stretches will make you a more productive worker, whatever you do for a living.

An everyday habit

Perseverance is simple when you make stretches an everyday habit. Habits can be formed in as little as 21 days, so set a goal on your calendar for the next 21 days and find opportunities for a stretch at home, work, and play. Have faith: the body will change, but only with persistence. Stretching in everyday life makes that persistence easy.

Take a twist break at the office. Cross one leg over the other and turn in the direction of the crossed leg, just as in our Seated cross-leg twist (see p.30).

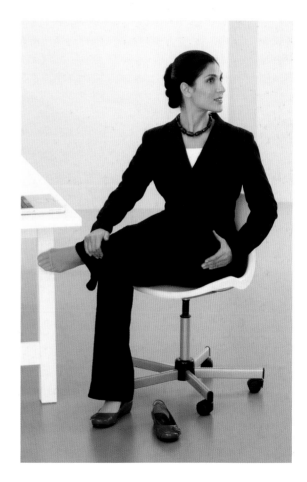

>> **relaxation** techniques

Relaxation takes discipline in a busy world. Chores, obligations, and crises sap your energy reserves and present road blocks to emotional balance. Try these scheduled and unscheduled calming techniques to make relaxation a priority in your life.

Relaxation is great for renewing the body, mind, and spirit. During every waking hour we expend our physical and mental energy, so we need to replenish it. Take a cue from professional athletes who aim for peak fitness. They know that the key to achieving optimal functioning lies in alternating periods of stress with times of relief and rest.

We all need a certain amount of stress in our lives to challenge and motivate us. But we also need to shake off any fatigue on a regular basis to avoid chronic weariness.

Sleep and rest

It's important for us all to renew our resources with nightly sleep and timely rest. Developing a healthy nightly ritual is essential in establishing an optimal renewal plan. Make your bedroom a sanctuary by creating a soothing, quiet place with your favourite

Use the contract–release method to lessen the tensions in your body. One by one, tighten and release each body part. End by tensing your whole body (inset, below), then let go and breathe deeply (main picture, below).

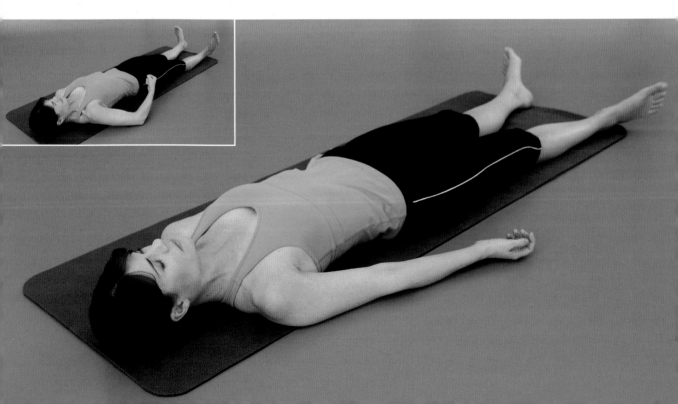

tips for dealing with daily stress

- **To cope with life's ups and downs** be sure to make time daily for refreshment and restoration.

- **Manage your stress**. Try a progressive relaxation technique, breathe deeply, or learn to meditate to reverse the effects of stress.

- **Develop good sleep hygiene**. Make your bedroom an inviting, quiet, peaceful sanctuary and let go of the day's hassles and worries.

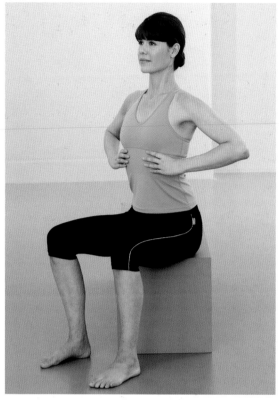

Practise deep breathing. The diaphragmatic breath is found by placing your fingers at the bottom of your breast bone and sniffing or coughing a few times. Inhale deeply; feel the rib cage expand.

bedding and gentle lighting. Don't have the television or your computer in the bedroom. It should be a space strictly for unwinding.

Don't drink alcohol last thing at night. Instead, savour a cup of a caffeine-free drink for an uninterrupted night's sleep. Some people find a warm bath before bed helps to relax them. Light reading material can also quieten the mind and help you leave the day's worries behind you. Make sure the room is completely dark while you're asleep. Studies have shown that exposure to light during sleep can disturb your body's natural cycles.

If you awaken during the night, focus on the pleasant texture of the bedding, take deep breaths, and relish the luxurious time you have for rest. Try to get seven to eight hours of the deep sleep you need for complete physical restoration.

Using stretching to help you relax

Relaxation techniques can greatly influence the restoration cycle. Simple exercises such as the progressive contract–relax technique (see opposite) can quickly lower body tension and take your mind away from over-analytical thoughts. For instance, tense the fists as you count to ten, then relax them. In order of progression, apply the same tense-then-relax method to the shoulders, thighs, calves, feet,

abdomen, and finally the face, puckering your lips and eyes strongly. End the technique by tensing your entire body, and then completely let go of all your body tension as you breathe five deep, long breaths. Notice how relaxed your body and your mind have become.

Another simple yet reliable relaxation technique, excellent for any setting and any location, is deep diaphragmatic breathing (see above). Place your fingers at the bottom of your breast bone to find the way your diaphragm moves. Sniff quickly several times or cough to feel the muscles move. Breathe into the diaphragm and feel these muscles expand for four seconds (think "1-alligator, 2-alligator", etc.). Then exhale for 8 seconds. Slow breathing reverses the fight-or-flight, adrenalin-based panic that's part of our fast-paced society.

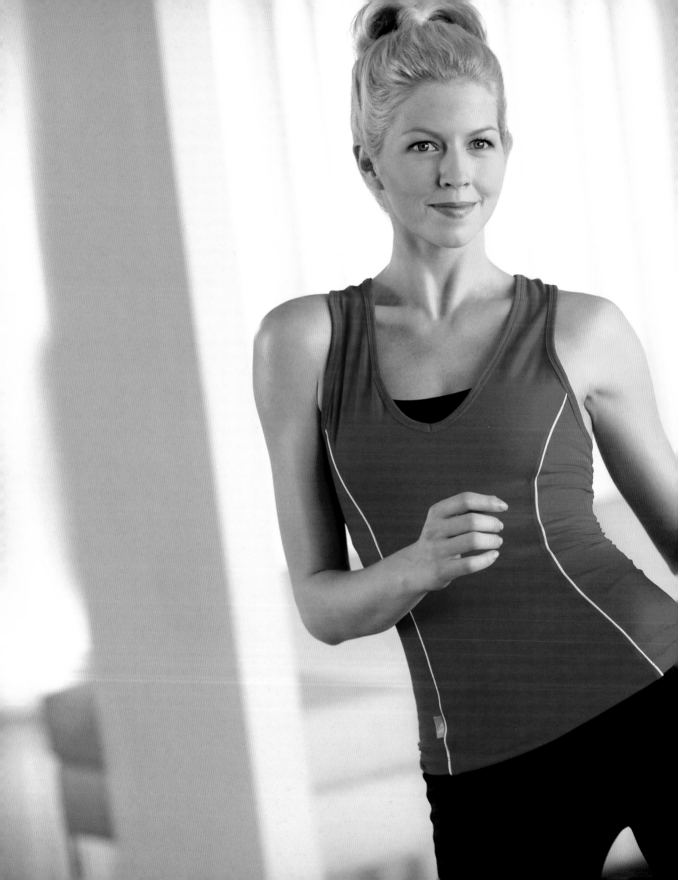

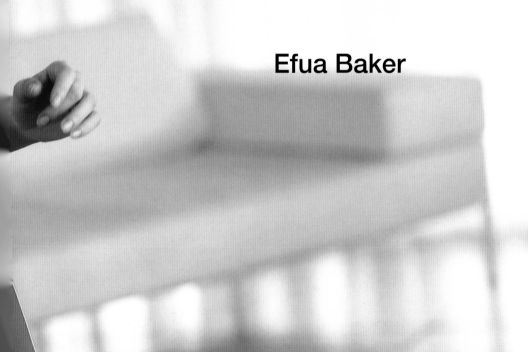

>> **15** minute

calorie burn

workout

Efua Baker

>> **what** are calories?

Calories are units of energy. They provide the fuel we need for our body to function – to keep our heart beating, for breathing, for digestion, for making new blood cells, and for maintaining our body temperature. They also provide us with the fuel for moving and exercising.

We get our calories from the food we eat, just as a car gets its power from petrol. Unfortunately, unlike a car, we don't have a limited amount of space – the petrol tank – to store fuel that isn't used immediately. Bodies are very accommodating. They will store any excess fuel (calories) in case of a famine. The problem is that this excess is stored in the form of fat around our bodies.

All we need to do, it seems, is to "balance the books". Take in roughly as much fuel as we use and – voilà – no spare fuel tanks required!

So how much energy *do* we use? To maintain a healthy body weight, women require an average of 2200 calories per day and men 2500 calories. But to find how much you need as an individual is not straightforward. Your Basal Metabolic Rate (BMR)

CALCULATING YOUR DAILY CALORIE REQUIREMENT

To work out your daily calorie requirement, you first need to find your Basal Metabolic Rate (BMR) – the amount of energy your body needs to maintain itself. This accounts for 50 to 80 per cent of your total energy use. The rest of the energy you need is for your muscles to work as you move in your daily life. That varies according to your level of activity and whether you are a man or a woman.
Note: 1in = 2.54cm; 1kg = 2.2lb

Men's BMR = 66 + (13.7 x weight in kg) + (5 x height in cm) – (6.8 x age in years)

Women's BMR = 655 + (9.6 x weight in kg) + (1.8 x height in cm) – (4.7 x age in years)
So if you're female, 30 years old, 167.6cm tall (5ft 6in), and weigh 54.5kg (120lb), your BMR =
655 + 523 + 302 – 141 = 1339 calories/day

Now that you know your BMR, you can work out your **daily calorie requirement** by using the chart below:
So if your BMR is 1339 calories per day, and you are moderately active, your daily calorie requirement =
1.55 x 1339 = 2075 calories/day

ACTIVITY LEVEL	BMR		
If you're sedentary (little or no exercise, desk job)	BMR	x	1.2
Gently active (light exercise/sports 1–3 days a week)	BMR	x	1.375
Moderately active (moderate exercise/sports 3–5 days a week)	BMR	x	1.55
Very active (hard exercise/sports 6–7 days a week)	BMR	x	1.725
Extra active (hard daily exercise/sports and physical job)	BMR	x	1.9

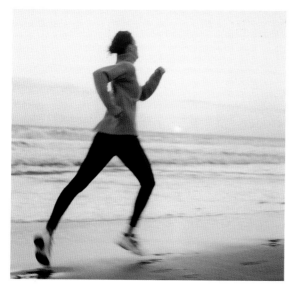

Going out for a run is a great way to burn calories and a chance to get out in the fresh air. You can run off a juicy 150 calories with just 15 minutes' running.

HOW MANY CALORIES CAN I BURN?

Whether you're exercising or simply doing household chores, you're always burning calories. This chart shows you how many, on average, a person weighing 70kg (155lb) burns doing each activity for 15 minutes. The calories burned vary according to your age, weight, level of fitness, and how hard you exercise.

DO THIS FOR 15 MINUTES	KCALS BURNED
Skipping with a rope	185
Boxing with a partner	165
Running (8kph/5mph)	150
Cross-country skiing	149
Cycling (20kph/12.5mph)	149
High-impact aerobics	130
Downhill skiing	111
Swimming	110
Shovelling snow	110
Low-impact aerobics	100
Dancing	100
Gardening	83
Childcare	65
Raking the lawn	60
Cooking	46
Sitting in a meeting	30
Working at the computer	26
Watching TV	14
Sleeping	11

is the amount of energy your body needs to function at rest, but we all burn/use calories at different rates. Your BMR is influenced by your age, sex, lean-muscle-to-fat ratio (a lean, muscular person will burn more calories than someone with a higher proportion of fat, even while sleeping), and your genetic package. The table opposite shows you how to calculate your daily calorie requirement. If you eat more than this, and don't move more, then you are simply going to get fat!

Let's say you want to lose 3.5kg (7lb). To get rid of just 0.5kg (1lb) of excess fat you must burn off around 3500 calories. Of course, you can pare down what you eat (and eating little and often also helps burn calories) but if you go for a two-pronged attack – diet *and* exercise – you have a much better chance of success. It's simple. Take in less fuel, burn more off. What is more, exercise will help build muscle which, in turn, will burn more fat.

So, what sort of exercise helps to burn the calories? Any exercise is better than none, but it's generally accepted that the best is aerobic exercise. This means working your cardiovascular system – the heart and lungs – by doing continuous, rhythmic exercise using large muscle

groups. All the sequences in this book are aerobic, so following them is the best place to start, but the chart above shows how many calories you can burn doing different forms of exercise.

As well as knowing how many calories I burn when I exercise, I also like to have an idea of the calorific value of the foods I eat. Eating a chocolate shortcake cookie means I need to do 15 minutes of low-impact aerobics to compensate. Hmmm ...

>> the **motivation** game

Different things motivate different people to get fit, so first and foremost, it's essential to find the key to start your engine! If you're not clear why exercise is important, read on and discover that, whatever your reasons for exercising, the benefits can't be beaten.

For most of the people I work with, looking good is the main reason they hire me as their body sculptor. This may be what motivates you, too, whether you're aiming for a bikini holiday, a wedding, or simply to have your friends remark on how great you're looking lately.

It's true that there are more important, health-related reasons for exercising (see opposite), but there's no denying that for a lot of people, physical appearance is their number one motivation. And that's OK. Because the positive side effects of exercising on a regular basis are manifold – you'll be looking and feeling better, because your body is becoming fitter and healthier.

Finding exercise you enjoy means you are more likely to stay motivated. Exercising with a friend helps, too. You wouldn't want to let your friend down, would you?

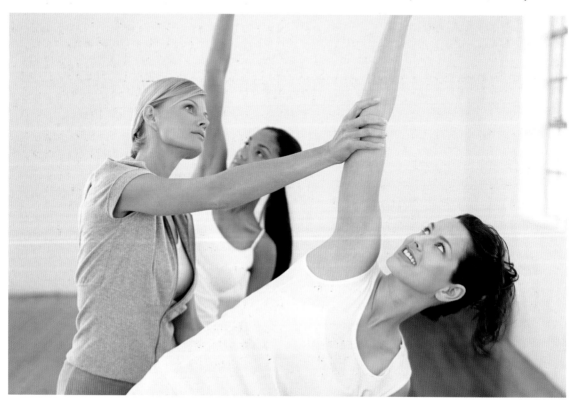

Then there's another category of people who turn to exercise because they're finding that things they could do without thinking 10 or 20 years ago are much harder. Suddenly, gardening, housework, or doing a favourite sport aren't as easy as they once were. For these people, exercise is a route to becoming strong and supple enough to carry on doing the things they've always done.

The health benefits

We all know more or less what we could be doing to benefit our bodies. Regular exercise promotes better cardiovascular and respiratory function. Studies have shown, beyond doubt, that it reduces the risks of coronary heart disease, lowers blood pressure, and also increases levels of "good" cholesterol. It can stabilize blood-sugar levels and so can prevent or control type II diabetes. It also improves bone density, which protects against osteoporosis. What is more, exercise can help delay some of the physiological effects of ageing and creates beneficial changes in the metabolism of the body, for instance speeding up the rate at which it burns calories (see p.102).

Additionally, exercise helps to combat sleep disorders such as insomnia, and it brings psychological benefits, too, for instance releasing stress and improving self-confidence. These days exercise is frequently prescribed for patients with depression, and can be as effective as some anti-depressant medications. On top of that, regular exercise is linked to better sexual function and an increased sex drive.

Working out regularly promotes stronger bones, flexible muscles, better posture and breathing function, and a generally more efficient body – all of which means you will look better. And we all know that it's easier to relate to results we can see, such as improved muscle tone or weight loss, than to "invisible" improvements in cholesterol, blood pressure, and bone-density levels. However, remember you will be reaping benefits in those areas, too, as a bonus, whether you are interested in them or not. So what on earth are you waiting for? Start exercising!

>> **top tips** to stay motivated

- **Find a form of exercise** you enjoy so you'll be sure to look forward to it. There are so many different types on offer, there's bound to be one for you.

- **Results are key**, so take advice (and read this book) to find out what exercise gives fast, lasting results. Once you see your body change for the better, it will reduce your chances of giving up.

- **Training for a particular event** is a great way to stay on track. Fun runs and mini triathlons are ideal for helping you to stay focused as you work towards the big day.

- **Keep your body on its toes.** Like you, your body loves variety, so make small changes in your workout from time to time. That keeps *you* interested and wakes your body up and helps it to burn more calories.

- **Stopped seeing results?** Change your programme, try a different class, or work with a different piece of equipment. Just as small changes in your workout can give your body a jump-start, so a complete change is as good as a full engine clean.

- **Use a personal trainer.** Seeing a personal trainer, even if it's just once or twice so they can design a personalized plan for you, can give you a boost and accelerate your progress once you are up and running.

- **Work with a friend.** If you train with an exercise buddy, you'll find it that much harder to skip a session than if you're home alone.

- **If finding even 15 minutes** a day is beyond you right now, work some extra activity into your life. Try gardening, walking part of the way to work, or cycling.

>> **personalize** your exercise

Your 15 Minute Calorie Burn Workout is hopefully just a start. Read on if you want to burn calories even faster or to learn how to tone things down if you're out of condition or are having an off-day. My tips show the way and – even better – they can be applied to almost any exercise.

If you're going to the trouble of taking 15 minutes out of your day to follow my workouts, then it makes sense to try to maximize your results. It's natural to ask how you can burn even more calories in 15 minutes, especially if you find it hard to resist the occasional sweet treat the rest of the time. Also, as you progress with your exercise, you may discover that you reach a "plateau" (see p.105). This is because your body cleverly adjusts to your level of work and decides to take a holiday. You need to give it a wake-up call from time to time.

You'll be glad to know that there are plenty of ways of intensifying your exercise, both to burn more calories in the time available and to get yourself off the "plateau".

Flawless form

Firstly, remind yourself to work with flawless form all the time. That means holding your tummy in, keeping your back straight, and keeping your shoulders relaxed. It's not as easy as it sounds, and it's precisely for that reason that you'll burn more calories. Think of the effort it takes just to keep your tummy in. That effort translates into more calories burned. Not only that, but working your muscles harder means that they become sleek and toned that much faster.

Practising a technique descriptively titled "mind to muscle" will help you work with flawless form. Simply focus on the area you want to feel working, and try to channel your muscle tension and effort on that area. At the same time make a conscious effort to relax any other part of your body you feel is trying to "join in". This may sound very simple, but if you master this technique you are without a doubt going to get a lot more out of your training.

Max your moves

Next, it pays to put all you've got into each move. When you're marching, lift your knees high and really swing your arms. If you're jogging, pick your

> ## >> **taking it** down a notch
>
> - **Go from high-impact to low-impact.** If you're doing the Jog (pp.138, 152), bring it down to the level of the March (pp.134, 152). If you're doing the Skip (p.116), do the March.
>
> - **Omit the hops and jumps.** If you're getting out of breath, simply take a step instead of doing a hop or a jump.
>
> - **Bring your arms down.** Raising your hands above your head increases your heart rate, so if it's getting too much, take them down and concentrate on maintaining good form and the footwork.
>
> - **Do your cool down stretches on the floor.** If you're exhausted at the end of a workout, don't skip your cool down, but stretch on the floor instead.

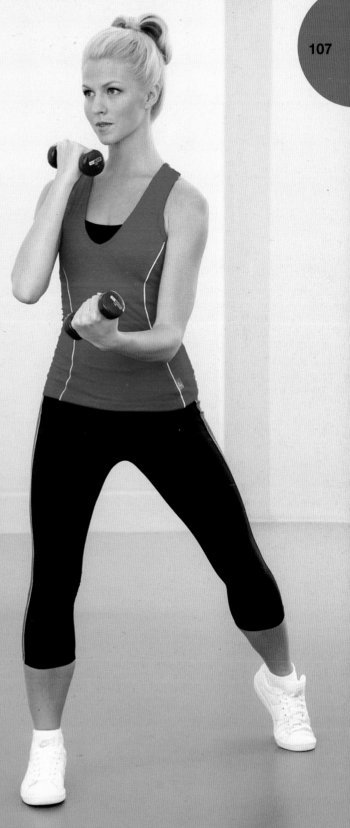

feet up and focus on springing off the floor. Intensify any side-to-side steps by making those steps bigger. Exaggerate all the up-down movements. Punch and kick with power. Any and all of these will burn off just a few extra calories and you'll quickly find that they add up.

Add some weight

Another tip is to get yourself a pair of small handweights and do the workouts holding those. If you find that awkward, you can wear weighted fingerless gloves instead. Start with a very light weight, say, 250g–500g (8oz–1lb) in/on each hand. Follow the workout and you'll be surprised how heavy those dinky little weights start to feel. Don't be put off by that. The weights are what make you work harder and burn calories faster. They will also give you fabulously toned arms. When you work with weights, be careful to maintain your form throughout, and if you can't manage that, then just put the weights down for a while.

Extend your workout

Last but not least, if you're prepared to work for more than your allotted 15 minutes, there's no reason – as long as you can still do the fitness test (see p.8) – why you can't lengthen your workout. You could double up on the number of reps you do for each step, you could repeat the entire workout again, from Step 9 to Step 18, or you could follow Step 9 to Step 18 from one workout with Step 9 to Step 18 from another. Just remember to always start with a warm up (Steps 1 to 8), and finish with a cool down (Steps 19 to 24).

Burn off extra calories by doing the routines holding handweights. The extra weight makes your body work harder, and you'll get fabulous arms at the same time.

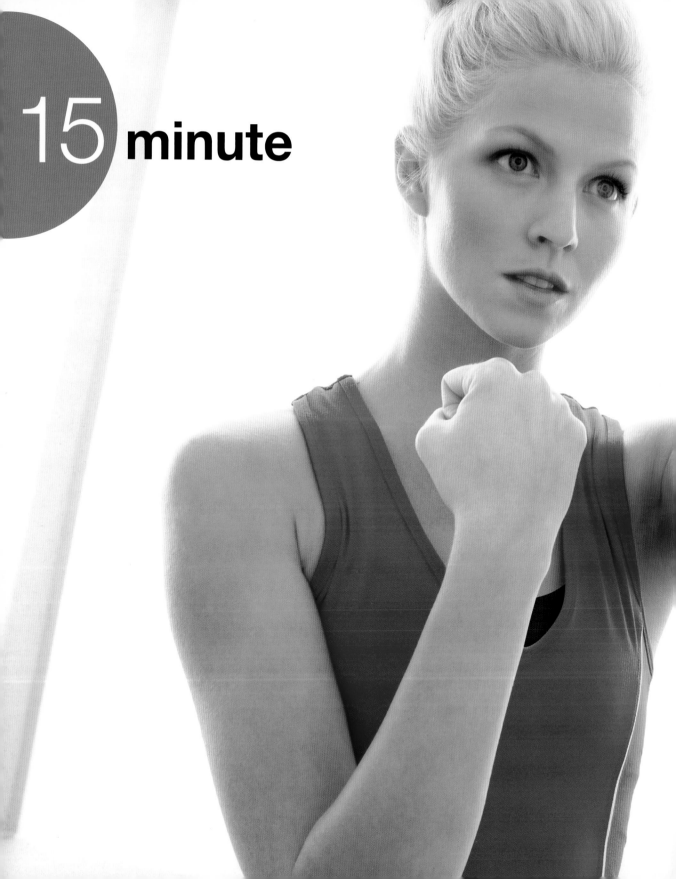

15 minute

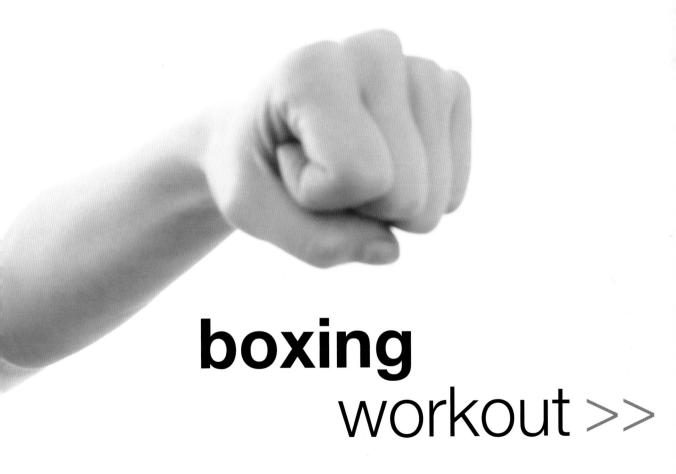

boxing
workout >>

Box your way to a leaner,
more powerful physique.
Strengthen and tone the
body. Focus the mind.

>> **boxing** workout

The various styles of boxing give the most intense all-over body training I have ever tried. This is one of the more demanding workouts in the book, blending the two styles – boxing and kickboxing. It's a great stress reliever, as well as a way of burning maximum calories during your 15 minutes.

Boxing and kickboxing are becoming increasingly popular, particularly with women. This type of exercise is fun but challenging. The aerobic element will help you to sculpt your body and burn calories, while the coordination, power, and balance that all types of boxing training offer are undeniably empowering and can be great for your self-confidence, too.

My workout includes kicking, punching, ducking, and skipping. It is not only one of the most effective for stripping off unwanted weight, but you'd be hard pushed to find a muscle group that this sequence doesn't work.

Let's start with your abs. Although my sequence doesn't include any traditional sit-ups, it offers a great abdominal workout. As long as you maintain good form and posture, and really work on keeping your tummy pulled in (without holding your breath), you can achieve more than you think.

The various kicks are also great for working the abs. Once you have engaged the abs – isolated them and got them working – imagine your legs are being lifted by them as if on puppet strings. That makes you work from your centre. It also helps relax the front of your thighs (the quads), which can take over and dominate if you're not careful.

The biceps and chest muscles will also get a good workout. While performing jabs and punches, you need to pay attention to keeping your shoulders down and relaxed. You're not trying to work your neck. Focus on the work of your biceps and chest muscles instead.

> >> **tips for** your boxing workout
>
> - **Maintain "mind to muscle" focus (see p.106).** When punching, focus on the biceps; when kicking, focus on your bottom and legs. Your abs should be "on" throughout.
>
> - **Mimic a proper skipping action,** making small circular movements with your hands as if you were turning a skipping rope. You'll know you're doing it correctly when you feel it in your biceps.
>
> - **This is a demanding workout,** but worth mastering. Practice makes perfect, so don't be discouraged when you start.

Remember, too, that it's a lot harder actually punching or kicking something than punching or kicking into space. So, you need to strike into the air as hard as you can to maintain an element of power in your arms and legs.

This workout is designed to burn calories and tone muscles, but you'll also improve your coordination and focus, and it's a fantastic way to let off steam!

Your boxing workout exercises many of your muscle groups, and encourages coordination of the body, while helping you to generate power and balance.

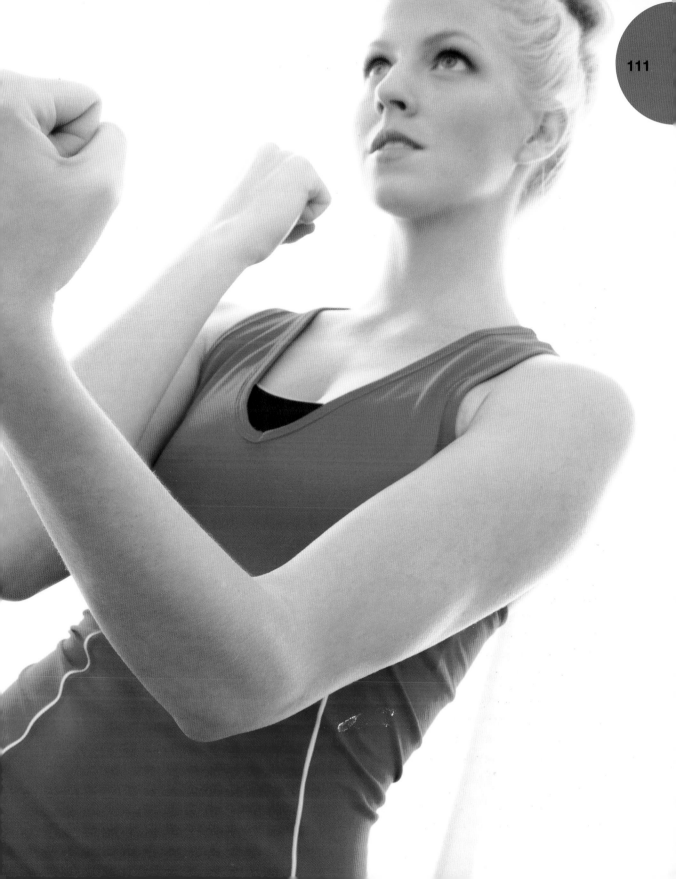

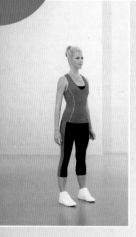

1 Stand tall with feet hip-width apart, knees soft, and arms by your sides. Relax your neck and shoulders, and make sure your tummy is pulled in. Take a deep breath in as you bend the knees and raise your arms above your head. Exhale as you lower them with a smooth circular movement. Make sure your back stays straight. Repeat for a total of 4 reps.

2 Alternate your weight from one foot to the other, rising up onto the ball of your foot. As you alternate feet, curl the opposite arm to your shoulder. Keep your hands in a loose fist and make sure you push your heel right down to the floor as you work your calf muscle. Repeat for a total of 16 reps (1 rep = both sides/directions).

to really lengthen your spine, lift from the hips as you raise the arms upwards

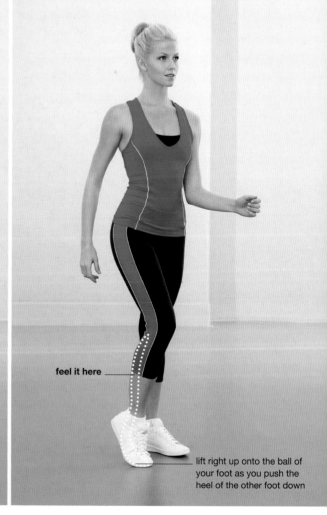

feel it here

lift right up onto the ball of your foot as you push the heel of the other foot down

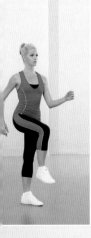

3 Standing on one foot, raise the other knee to waist-height. At the same time, raise the opposite arm. March on the spot, raising opposite knees and arms. Repeat for a total of 8 reps. Then, with your arms by your sides, raise your shoulders towards your ears and roll them in a circular motion, backwards, then forwards. Repeat for a total of 4 reps.

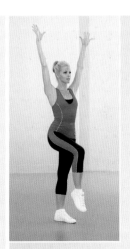

4 Continue marching and, as you do so, stretch your arms sideways to meet above your head, opening and closing your hands at intervals with a "flicking" motion, to warm your fingers and wrists. Continue "flicking" your hands as you lower your arms. Repeat for a total of 4 reps.

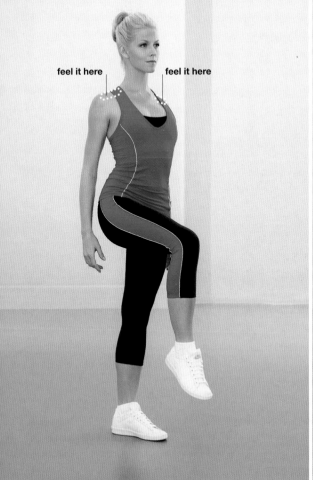

feel it here feel it here

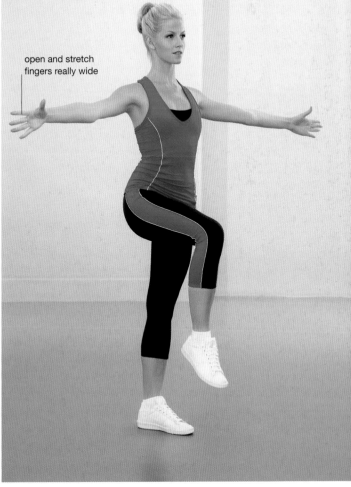

open and stretch fingers really wide

>> side step/back step

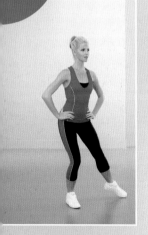

5 With hands on hips, take a step to one side, then bring your feet together. Repeat to the other side. Repeat for a total of 4 reps, then swing your arms in the same direction as you are stepping. Your arms should be relaxed and raised no higher than shoulder-height. Repeat for a total of 8 reps.

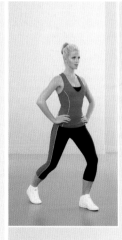

6 With hands on hips, touch one foot on the floor behind you. Return to centre and repeat with the opposite foot. Keep your weight centred as you alternate legs. Repeat for a total of 4 reps, then add an arm push in time with your leg movements by pushing both arms forward and back just below shoulder-height. Repeat for a total of 8 reps.

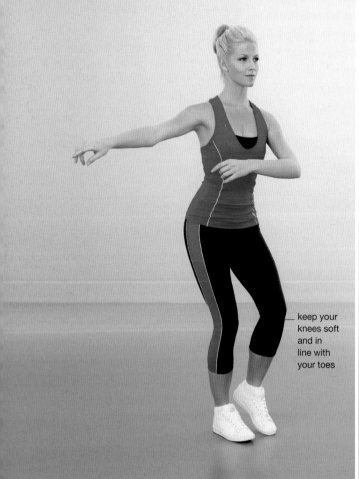

keep your knees soft and in line with your toes

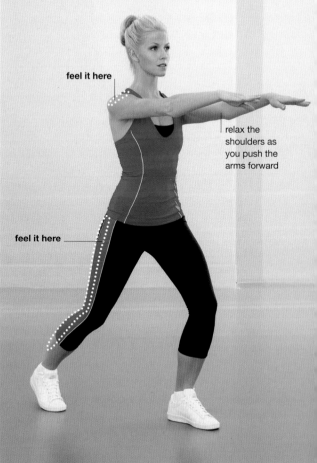

feel it here

relax the shoulders as you push the arms forward

feel it here

>> dip-kick with twist/roll-up

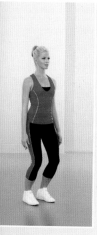

7 With arms by your sides, bend both knees, then come up and kick one foot forward. Repeat for a total of 8 reps, then add a twist by turning your upper body and swinging the opposite arm to the kicking leg. Keep the arms shoulder-height. Keep your hips square. Repeat, alternating sides, for a total of 8 reps.

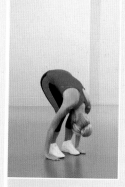

8 Stand tall with feet hip-width apart, arms stretched above your head, shoulders relaxed, and neck and spine in line. Slowly lower your arms and take your chin towards your chest, then round your back and slowly bend down towards the floor. When you are as low as possible, your hands should be relaxed and as near to the floor as is comfortable. Take a deep breath into your lower back. Then, keeping your tummy pulled into your lower back, uncurl slowly, one vertebra at a time, until you have returned to a standing position.

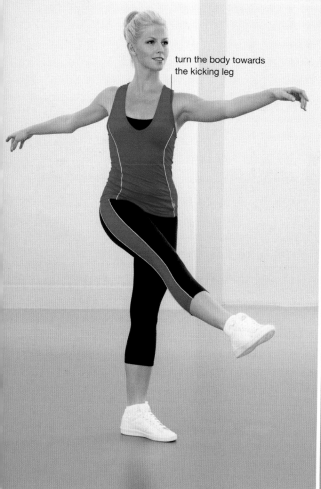

turn the body towards the kicking leg

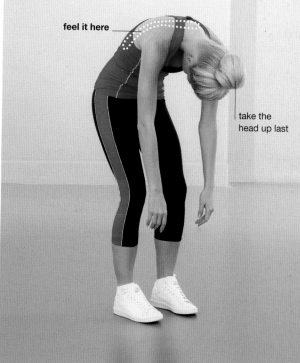

feel it here

take the head up last

>> punch across/skip

9 Standing with your feet slightly wider than hip-width apart, knees soft and pointing forward, punch one arm across your body for a total of 8 times, keeping the other fist tucked under your chin. Punch with the fist facing down. Repeat on the opposite side then, keeping your lower body in the same position, punch across your body, alternating sides for a total of 8 reps.

10 Bring your feet together, arms by your sides, and "skip" with an imaginary rope, alternating feet. Come up onto the balls of your feet as you lift your feet very slightly off the floor. As you "skip", make a small circular motion with your hands, as if you were turning the rope. Repeat for a total of 32 skips.

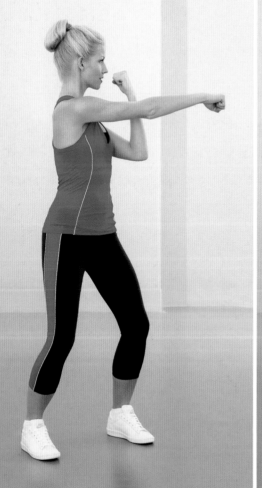

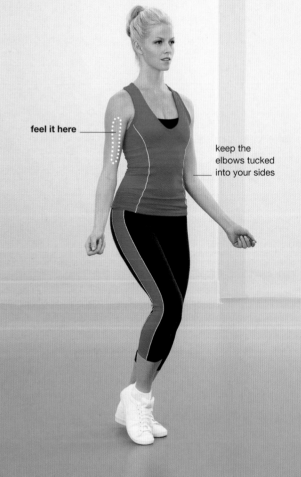

feel it here

keep the elbows tucked into your sides

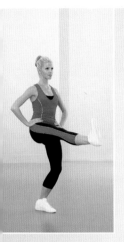

11 Starting with both feet together and hands on hips, kick one leg forward to hip-height, leading with the heel and flexing the foot. Return that leg behind to come into a lunge position resting on the toes. Repeat, making sure you keep your hips square and your knees always in line with your toes. Keep your tummy pulled in and your spine straight. Repeat for a total of 8 times, then change sides and repeat for a total of 8 times.

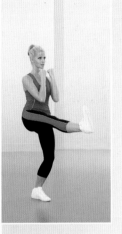

12 Starting with your feet together and both hands held as fists under your chin, kick one leg forward to hip-height, leading with the heel and flexing the foot. As you return that leg behind you to rest it on its toes, punch the opposite arm across the body at chest-height. Repeat for a total of 8 times, then change sides and repeat for a total of 8 times. Repeat Step 10.

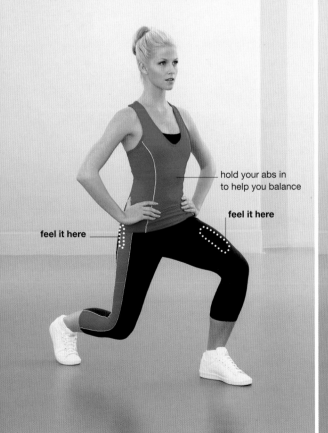

hold your abs in to help you balance

feel it here

feel it here

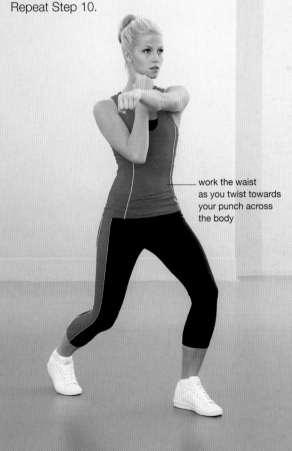

work the waist as you twist towards your punch across the body

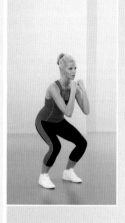

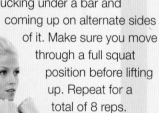

13 Starting with your feet hip-width apart, hands in fists under your chin, squat down. Keep your weight in your heels. Straighten your knees and come to standing, leaning to one side with the opposite heel coming off the floor. Squat down again and lift up on the other side. Imagine you are ducking under a bar and coming up on alternate sides of it. Make sure you move through a full squat position before lifting up. Repeat for a total of 8 reps.

14 Starting with your feet hip-width apart and both hands held as fists under your chin, squat down. Make sure your weight is in your heels. Then unbend your knees and come to standing, kicking out to the side with one leg. Lead with the heel and flex the foot. Repeat for a total of 4 times, returning to the centre squat position between each kick. Change sides and repeat for a total of 4 times. Repeat.

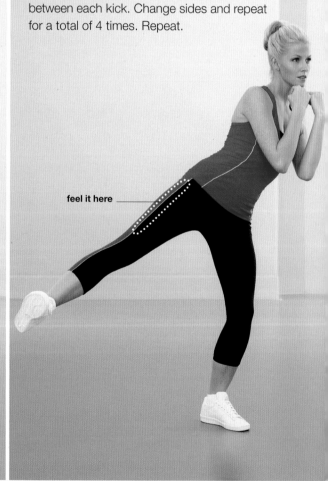

feel it here

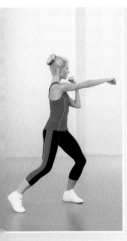

15 Starting with your feet hip-width apart and both hands held as fists under your chin, double-punch one arm across your body at chest-height, keeping the other fist under your chin. First punch with the fist facing the floor, then turn the arm and punch upwards. Twist your upper torso in the direction of the punch, lifting the opposite heel off the floor. Repeat on the other side. Repeat for a total of 8 reps. Repeat Step 10.

16 Starting with your feet together and both hands held as fists under your chin, kick one leg forward to hip-height, leading with the heel and flexing the foot. Keep the supporting leg slightly bent, and make sure the kicking foot returns parallel to the supporting leg. Repeat for a total of 8 times, then change sides and repeat for a total of 8 times. Repeat.

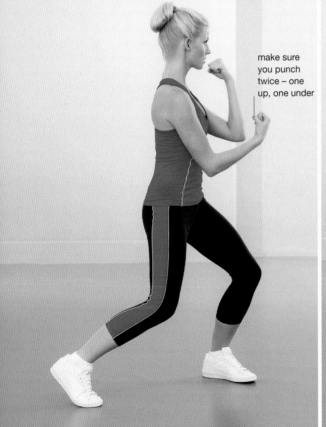

make sure you punch twice – one up, one under

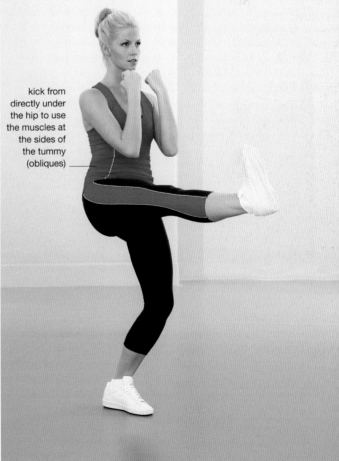

kick from directly under the hip to use the muscles at the sides of the tummy (obliques)

>> **arm roll/bent-over twist**

17 Marching on the spot and with elbows at chest-height and shoulders relaxed, roll your forearms over each other in a circular motion. Roll them as fast as you can while you count to 16, then change direction for another count of 16.

18 Position your feet wide and parallel, and with your knees slightly bent, bend at the waist to touch one hand to the outside of the opposite foot. As you touch, raise the other arm, keeping the elbow bent and pointing to the ceiling. Repeat, alternating sides, for a total of 16 reps.

Repeat Step 10, then Steps 9–12, then Step 10 again, then Steps 13–15, then Step 10 again, then Steps 16–18, and finally, Step 10 again.

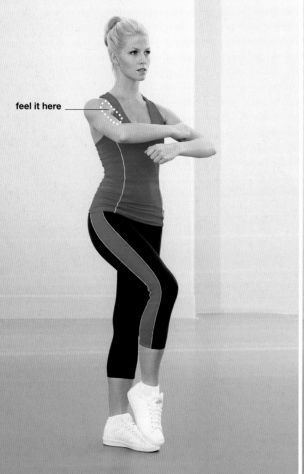

feel it here

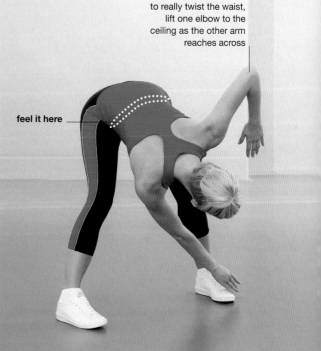

to really twist the waist, lift one elbow to the ceiling as the other arm reaches across

feel it here

19 Standing on one foot, raise the other knee to hip-height. At the same time, raise the opposite arm. March on the spot, raising opposite knees and arms. Repeat for a total of 24 reps.

20 Keeping both toes pointing forward, take one leg behind you, and bend the front knee. Clasp your hands in front and raise your arms towards your ears as you lower your head. You should feel a stretch in your upper back, neck, and calf.

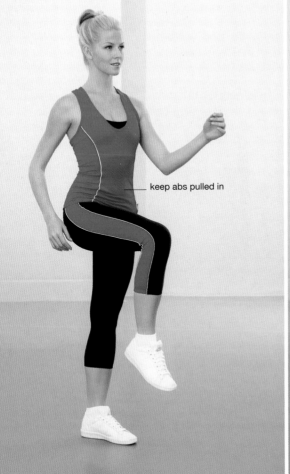

keep abs pulled in

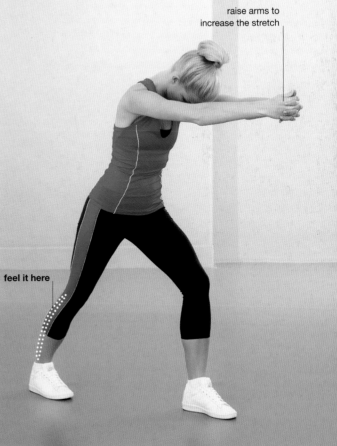

raise arms to increase the stretch

feel it here

>> 3-in-1 stretch 2/quad stretch

21 Position the other leg behind, toes pointing forward, and front knee bent. Clasp your hands behind your back. Open your chest as you raise your arms behind you. You should feel a stretch in your calf, chest, and arms.

22 Stand on one leg and hold the other foot with the hand on the same side. Bring the heel of the raised foot towards the buttock until you feel a stretch in the front of the bent-leg thigh. Change legs. If you cannot keep your balance, hold onto a support.

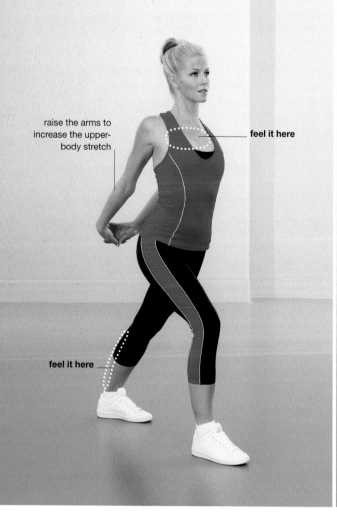

raise the arms to increase the upper-body stretch

feel it here

feel it here

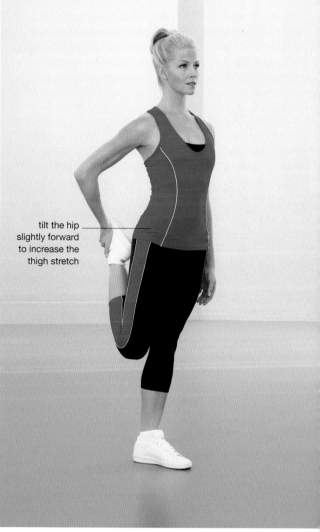

tilt the hip slightly forward to increase the thigh stretch

23 Take a step to one side and bend that knee, keeping the knee directly over the toes. Take your hands to the bent-leg thigh and lean forward, stretching the other leg out to the side. Make sure your neck and spine stay in line, and keep your back long and straight. You should feel a stretch in the inner thigh of the outstretched leg. Repeat on the other side.

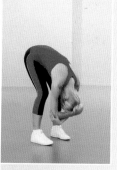

24 Stand tall with feet hip-width apart, arms stretched above your head, shoulders relaxed, and neck and spine in line. Slowly lower your arms and take your chin towards your chest, then round your back and slowly bend down towards the floor. When you are as low as possible, your hands should be relaxed and as near to the floor as is comfortable. Take a deep breath into your lower back. Then, keeping your tummy pulled into your lower back, uncurl slowly, one vertebra at a time, until you have returned to a standing position.

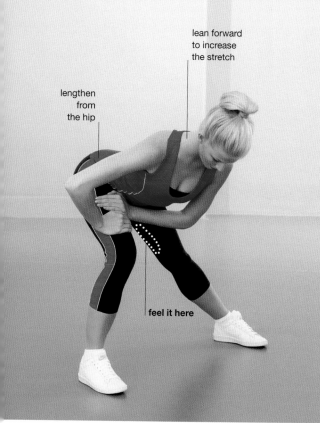

lengthen from the hip

lean forward to increase the stretch

feel it here

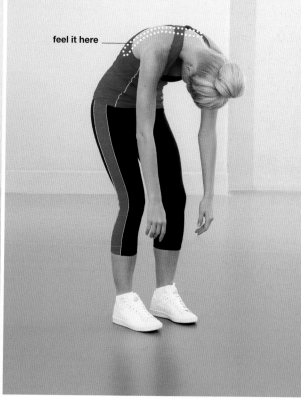

feel it here

boxing workout at a glance

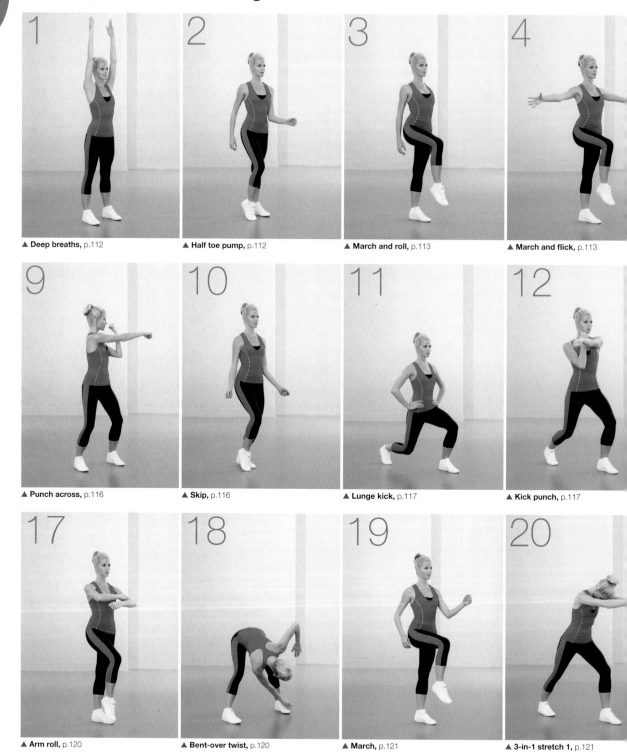

▲ **Deep breaths,** p.112

▲ **Half toe pump,** p.112

▲ **March and roll,** p.113

▲ **March and flick,** p.113

▲ **Punch across,** p.116

▲ **Skip,** p.116

▲ **Lunge kick,** p.117

▲ **Kick punch,** p.117

▲ **Arm roll,** p.120

▲ **Bent-over twist,** p.120

▲ **March,** p.121

▲ **3-in-1 stretch 1,** p.121

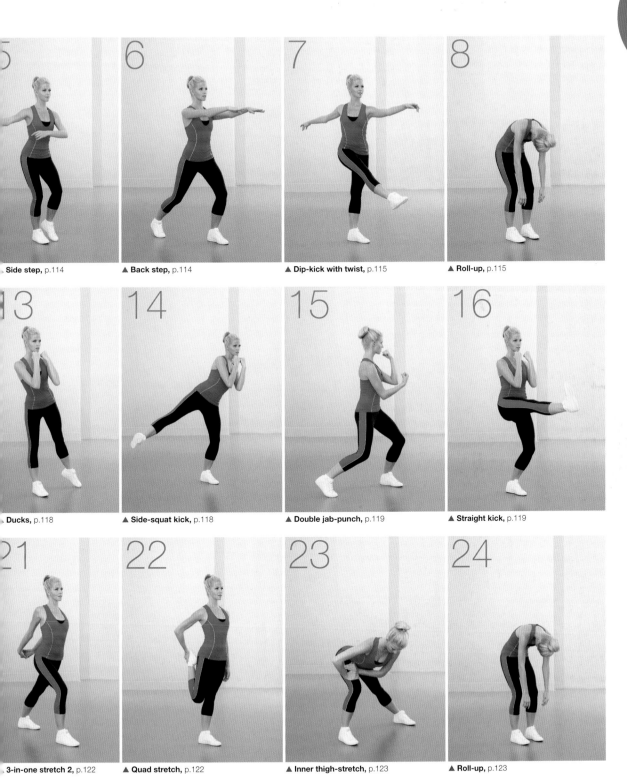

5 ▲ Side step, p.114

6 ▲ Back step, p.114

7 ▲ Dip-kick with twist, p.115

8 ▲ Roll-up, p.115

13 ▲ Ducks, p.118

14 ▲ Side-squat kick, p.118

15 ▲ Double jab-punch, p.119

16 ▲ Straight kick, p.119

21 ▲ 3-in-one stretch 2, p.122

22 ▲ Quad stretch, p.122

23 ▲ Inner thigh-stretch, p.123

24 ▲ Roll-up, p.123

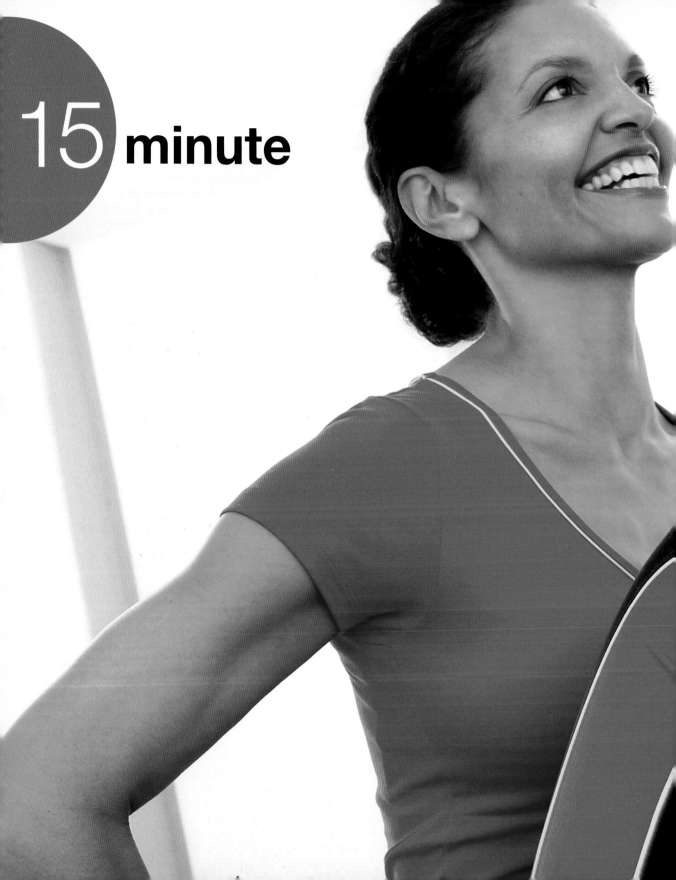

15 minute

aerobics
workout >>

Step, march, hop, jump! Raise your heart rate and your spirit as you exercise the old school way!

>> aerobics workout

Think of an aerobics workout and the chances are you'll conjure up an image of a class involving women wearing headbands and a lot of Lycra. That's how things were in the 1980s. This sequence offers you my collection of classic aerobic moves. Headbands and Lycra are optional!

The term "aerobics" was first used to describe a system of exercise which an exercise physiologist designed to help prevent heart disease. The system involved doing continuous, rhythmic activity using large muscle groups. In fact, all the sequences in my *15 Minute Calorie Burn Workout* are "aerobic", which is why they help you to burn calories.

The aerobics classes most of us recognize today have evolved from what started out in the US in the early 1970s and grew into a worldwide craze that became one of the defining features of the 1980s. If you happened to be around then – as I was – you may recall the hype that surrounded these particular classes. The combination of exercise, music, and the social aspect often proved irresistible. And because you could – and still can – work more or less intensively, depending on your ability, one of the advantages of aerobics classes was that they gave people of different fitness levels the chance to work together and have fun.

My own aerobics workout offers you the chance to do a collection of some classic – what I would call "vintage" – aerobic steps from the early days. Some of the moves, such as the Grapevine, Toe tap, and Rocking horse, were around then, and are often found in classes today.

Many of the steps in this aerobics workout are very simple, so it is important to monitor how hard you are training. Ideally, you should aim to work at a level where you are not too comfortable. If the steps feel easy to you, follow the tips on pages 106–107 to intensify your work rate.

> **>> tips for** your aerobics workout
>
> - In Chest march, you have to really relax the shoulders and arms to isolate the chest muscles properly. Your elbows should meet (or nearly meet) as you flex the chest.
>
> - In Side-dig swing, don't transfer all your weight to the foot you step out on. Keep your weight centred and "bounce" the step more. This helps you to keep in time.
>
> - In high-impact steps such as Crossover jump, be sure to land correctly, flexing your knees and rolling through your feet. Do it safely and don't rush it.

However, some of the steps – for example, Chest march, Side-dig swing, and Crossover jump – need your special attention (see above). And remember: quality is always more important than quantity.

Although you will be doing this workout in the comfort of your own home, imagine yourself in a 1980s class. Let yourself go and have fun. Perform the moves with enthusiasm. You could even get the rest of your family involved!

One of the benefits of doing a regular aerobics workout is that you can perform the steps with an intensity that suits you, and still burn the calories.

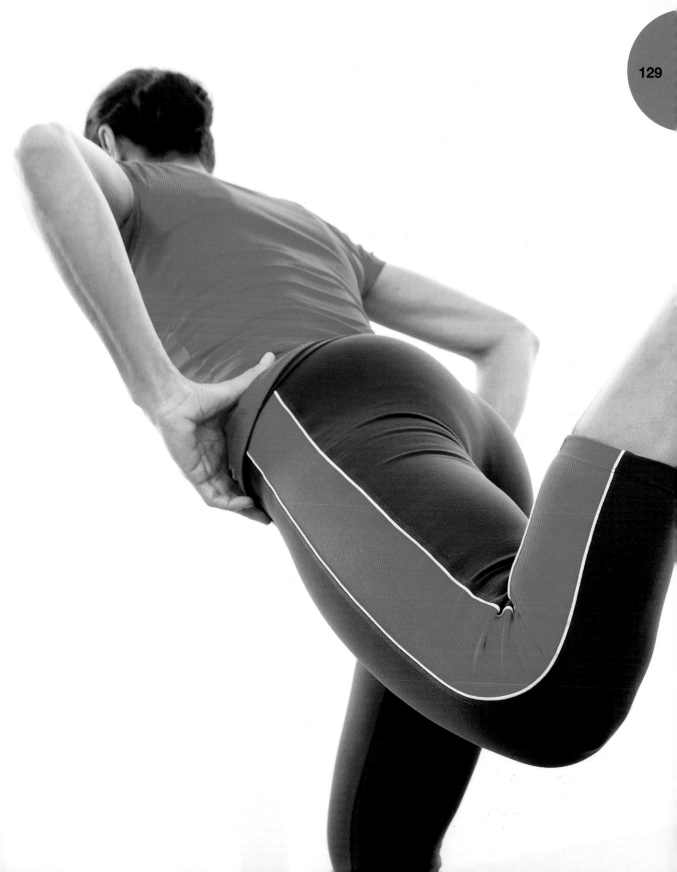

>> **deep breaths/half-toe pump**

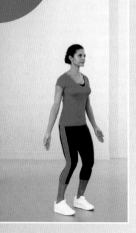

1 Stand tall with feet hip-width apart, knees soft, and arms by your sides. Relax your neck and shoulders, and make sure your tummy is pulled in. Take a deep breath in as you bend the knees and raise your arms above your head. Exhale as you lower them with a smooth circular movement. Make sure your back stays straight. Repeat for a total of 4 reps.

2 Alternate your weight from one foot to the other, rising up onto the ball of your foot. As you alternate feet, curl the opposite arm to your shoulder. Keep your hands in a loose fist and make sure you push your heel right down to the floor as you work your calf muscle. Repeat for a total of 16 reps (1 rep = both sides/directions).

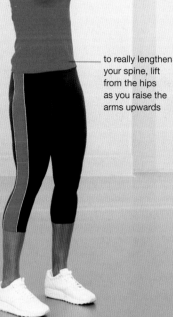

to really lengthen your spine, lift from the hips as you raise the arms upwards

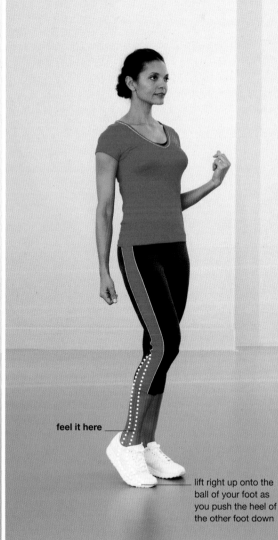

feel it here

lift right up onto the ball of your foot as you push the heel of the other foot down

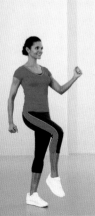

3 Standing on one foot, raise the other knee to waist-height. At the same time, raise the opposite arm. March on the spot, raising opposite knees and arms. Repeat for a total of 8 reps. Then, with your arms by your sides, raise your shoulders towards your ears and roll them in a circular motion, backwards, then forward. Repeat for a total of 4 reps.

4 Continue marching and, as you do so, stretch your arms sideways to meet above your head, opening and closing your hands at intervals with a "flicking" motion, to warm your fingers and wrists. Continue "flicking" your hands as you lower your arms. Repeat for a total of 4 reps.

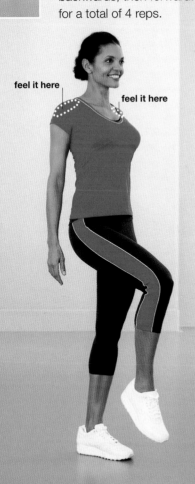

feel it here

feel it here

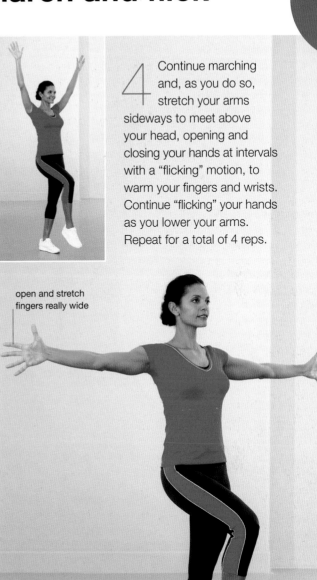

open and stretch fingers really wide

>> side step/back step

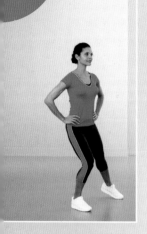

5 With hands on hips, take a step to one side, then bring your feet together. Repeat on the other side. Repeat for a total of 4 reps, then swing your arms in the same direction as you are stepping. Your arms should be relaxed and raised no higher than shoulder-height. Repeat for a total of 8 reps.

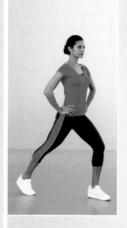

6 With hands on hips, touch one foot on the floor behind you. Return to centre. Repeat with the opposite foot. Keep your weight centred as you alternate legs. Repeat for a total of 4 reps, then add an arm push in time with your leg movements by pushing both arms forward and back just below shoulder-height. Repeat for a total of 8 reps.

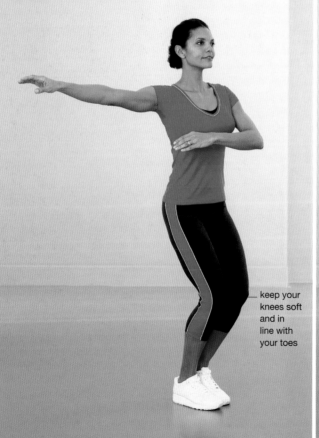

keep your knees soft and in line with your toes

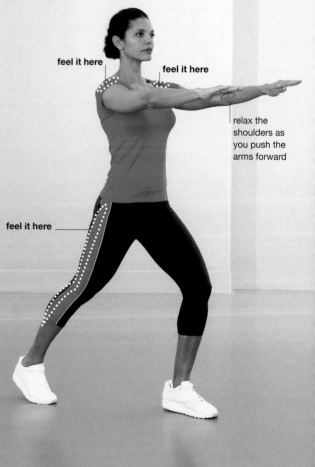

feel it here

feel it here

relax the shoulders as you push the arms forward

feel it here

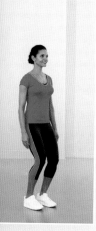

>> dip-kick with twist/roll-up

7 With arms by your sides, bend both knees, then come up and kick one foot forward. Repeat for a total of 8 reps, then add a twist by turning your upper body and swinging the opposite arm to the kicking leg. Keep your arms at shoulder-height and hips square. Repeat, alternating sides, for a total of 8 reps.

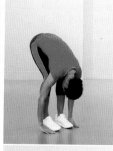

8 Stand tall with feet hip-width apart, arms stretched above your head, shoulders relaxed, and neck and spine in line. Slowly lower your arms and take your chin towards your chest, then round your back and slowly bend down towards the floor. When you are as low as possible, your hands should be relaxed and as near to the floor as is comfortable. Take a deep breath into your lower back. Then, keeping your tummy pulled into your lower back, uncurl slowly, one vertebra at a time, until you have returned to a standing position.

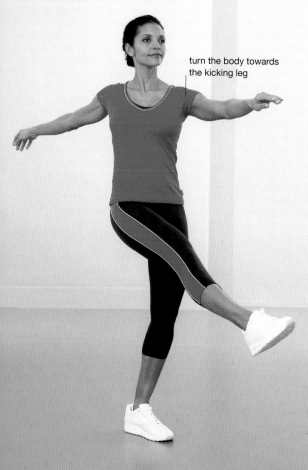

turn the body towards the kicking leg

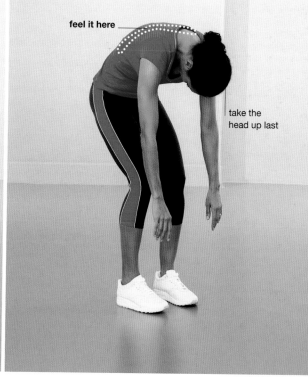

feel it here

take the head up last

>> toe tap/march

9 Standing with feet apart and knees slightly turned out, tap the toes of one foot on the floor to the side. As you tap, curl your arms at the elbow, alternating arms. Repeat for a total of 16 reps, then change feet and repeat for a total of 16 reps.

10 Standing on one foot, raise the other knee to waist-height. At the same time, raise the opposite arm. March on the spot, raising opposite knees and arms together. Repeat for a total of 16 reps.

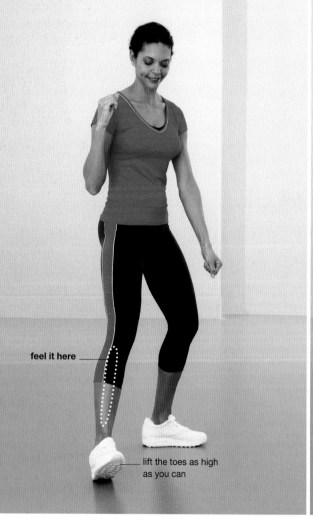

feel it here

lift the toes as high as you can

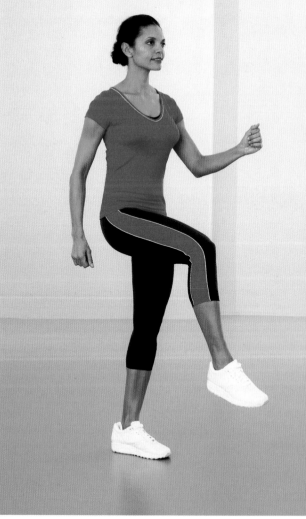

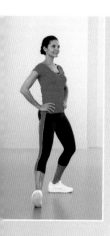

11 With hands on hips, step to the side, take the other foot behind, step to the side again, then bring the feet together. Repeat on the other side. Repeat for a total of 4 reps.

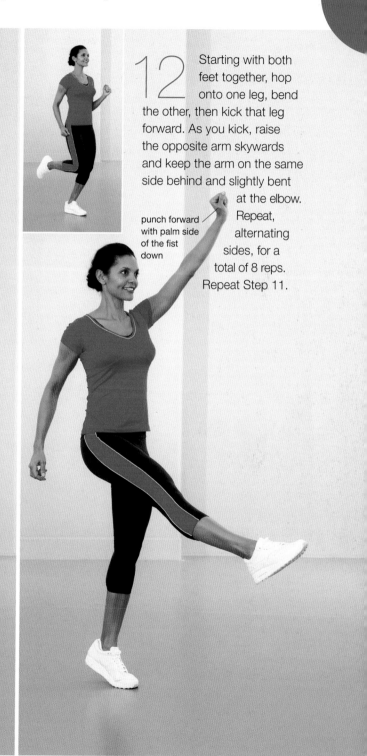

12 Starting with both feet together, hop onto one leg, bend the other, then kick that leg forward. As you kick, raise the opposite arm skywards and keep the arm on the same side behind and slightly bent at the elbow. Repeat, alternating sides, for a total of 8 reps. Repeat Step 11.

punch forward with palm side of the fist down

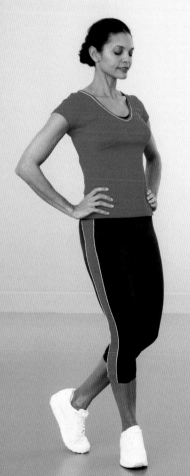

>> crossover jump/chest march

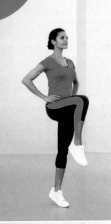

13 Starting with both feet together and hands on hips, jump, taking one knee to hip-height. Cross that leg over the other, touching the toe briefly to the floor. Bring the knee back to hip-height, then back to centre. Repeat on the other side. Repeat for a total of 8 reps.

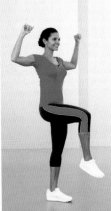

14 Standing on one foot, raise the other knee to hip-height and take the arms to the sides at shoulder-height, elbows bent. March on the spot, bringing the elbows together at chest-height, then opening them. Repeat for a total of 16 times.

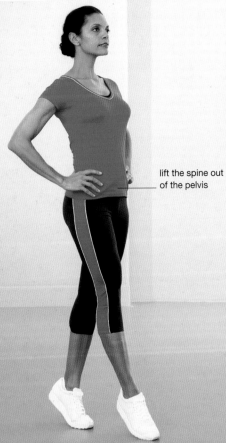

lift the spine out of the pelvis

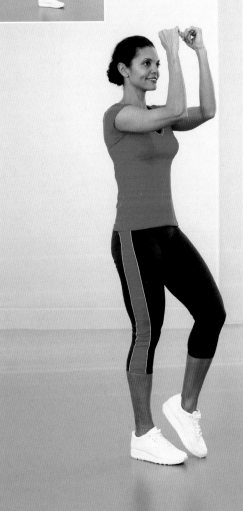

>> rocking horse/side-dig swing

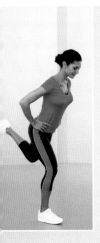

15 Starting with both feet together and hands on hips, step forward onto one foot and bend the other leg behind at the knee. Rock slightly onto the front leg. Step the back leg down, raise the front leg and rock slightly onto the back leg. Repeat the forward and back rocking motion for a total of 8 reps. Change sides and repeat for a total of 8 reps. Repeat Step 11.

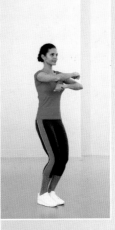

16 Starting with both feet together and arms in front of you at chest-height with elbows bent, step to one side. As you step, open the arms to the sides, elbows still bent. Bring the feet and arms together, then step to the other side and open the arms again. Repeat, alternating sides, for a total of 8 reps.

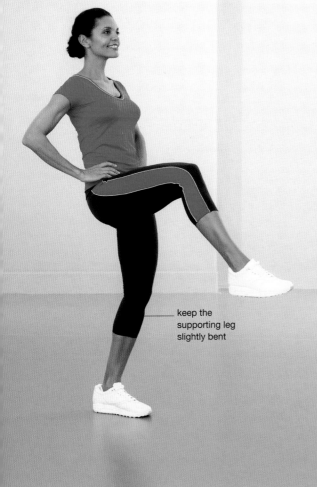

keep the supporting leg slightly bent

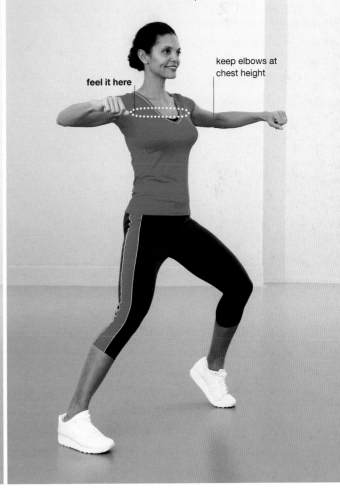

feel it here

keep elbows at chest height

>> **jog/cross-country ski**

17 Curling the opposite arm to the lifted knee, jog on the spot, raising your heels towards your buttocks. Make sure your heels touch the ground every time you land. Repeat for a total of 16 reps.

18 Standing on one leg, take the arm on the same side up and forward and take the other leg behind. The other arm stays by your side. Keeping the knees bent, change sides. Repeat, alternating sides, for a total of 4 reps. Make sure you work from your centre, keeping your tummy pulled in for good balance.

Repeat Step 11, then Steps 9–12, then Step 11 again, then Steps 13–15, then Step 11 again, then Steps 16–18, then Step 11 again, then Steps 9–12, then Step 11 again, then Steps 13–15, then Step 11 again, then Steps 16–18, and finally, Step 11 again.

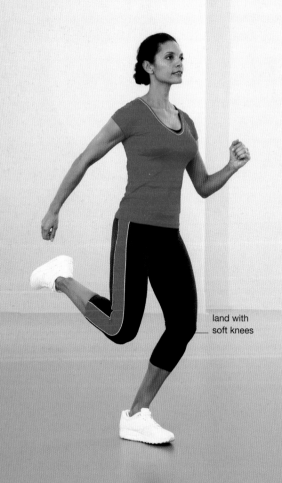

land with
soft knees

feel it here

feel it here

19 Standing on one foot, raise the other knee to hip-height. At the same time, raise the opposite arm. March on the spot, raising opposite knees and arms. Repeat for a total of 24 reps.

20 Keeping both toes pointing forward, take one leg behind you, and bend the front knee. Clasp your hands in front and raise your arms towards your ears as you lower your head. You should feel a stretch in your upper back, neck, and calf.

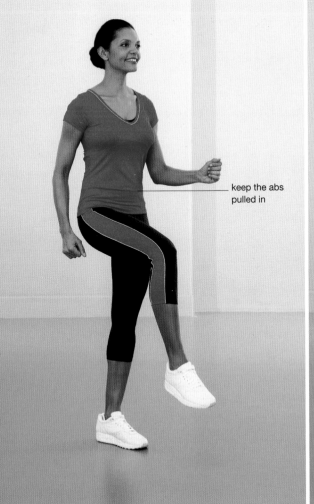

keep the abs pulled in

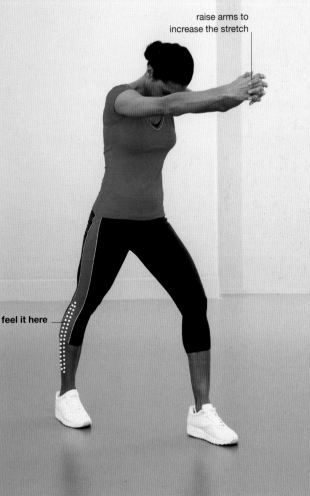

raise arms to increase the stretch

feel it here

>> 3-in-1 stretch 2/quad stretch

21 Take the other leg behind, toes pointing forward, and front knee bent. Clasp your hands behind your back. Open your chest as you raise your arms behind you. You should feel a stretch in your calf, chest, and arms.

22 Stand on one leg and hold the other foot with the hand on the same side. Bring the heel of the raised foot towards the buttock until you feel a stretch in the front of the bent-leg thigh. Change legs. If you cannot keep your balance, hold onto a support.

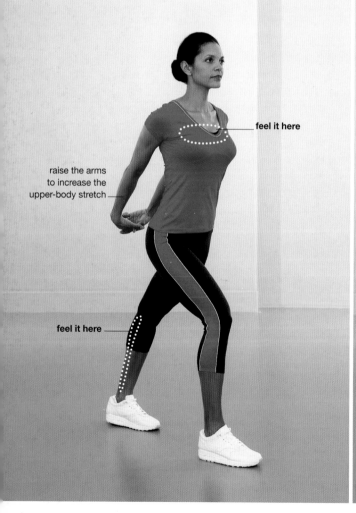

feel it here

raise the arms to increase the upper-body stretch

feel it here

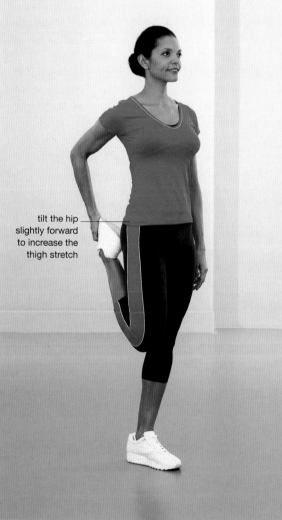

tilt the hip slightly forward to increase the thigh stretch

23 Take a step to one side and bend that knee, keeping the knee directly over the toes. Take your hands to the bent-leg thigh and lean forward, stretching the other leg out to the side. Make sure your neck and spine stay in line, and keep your back long and straight. You should feel a stretch in the inner thigh of the outstretched leg. Repeat on the other side.

24 Stand tall with feet hip-width apart, arms stretched above your head, shoulders relaxed, and the neck and spine in line. Slowly lower your arms and take your chin towards your chest, then round your back and slowly bend down towards the floor. When you are as low as possible, your hands should be relaxed and as near to the floor as is comfortable. Take a deep breath into your lower back. Then, keeping your tummy pulled into your lower back, uncurl slowly, one vertebra at a time, until you have returned to a standing position.

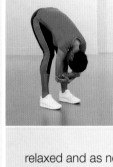

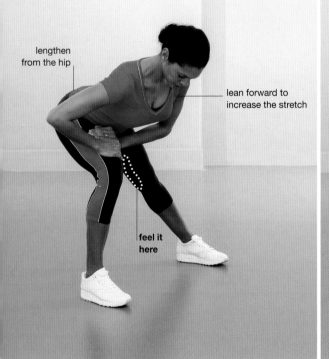

lengthen from the hip

lean forward to increase the stretch

feel it here

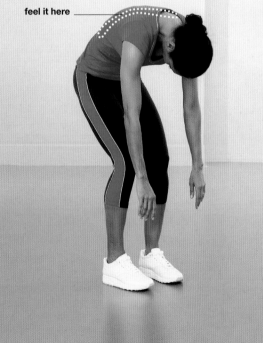

feel it here

aerobic workout at a glance

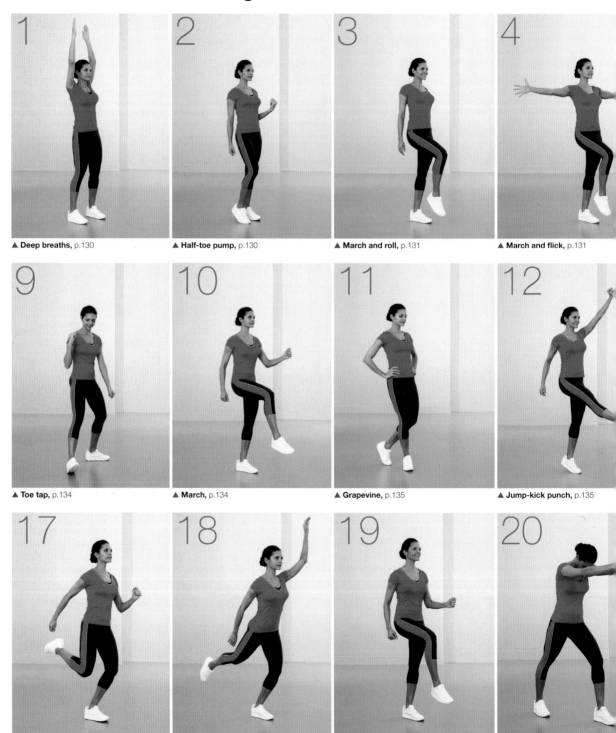

▲ **Deep breaths,** p.130

▲ **Half-toe pump,** p.130

▲ **March and roll,** p.131

▲ **March and flick,** p.131

▲ **Toe tap,** p.134

▲ **March,** p.134

▲ **Grapevine,** p.135

▲ **Jump-kick punch,** p.135

▲ **Jog,** p.138

▲ **Cross-country ski,** p.138

▲ **March,** p.139

▲ **3-in-1 stretch 1,** p.139

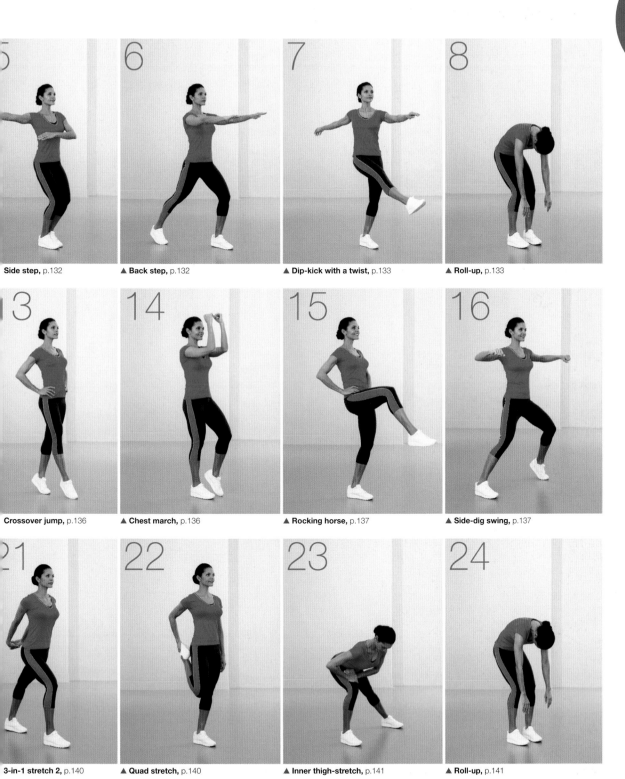

5 Side step, p.132

6 ▲ Back step, p.132

7 ▲ Dip-kick with a twist, p.133

8 ▲ Roll-up, p.133

13 Crossover jump, p.136

14 ▲ Chest march, p.136

15 ▲ Rocking horse, p.137

16 ▲ Side-dig swing, p.137

21 3-in-1 stretch 2, p.140

22 ▲ Quad stretch, p.140

23 ▲ Inner thigh-stretch, p.141

24 ▲ Roll-up, p.141

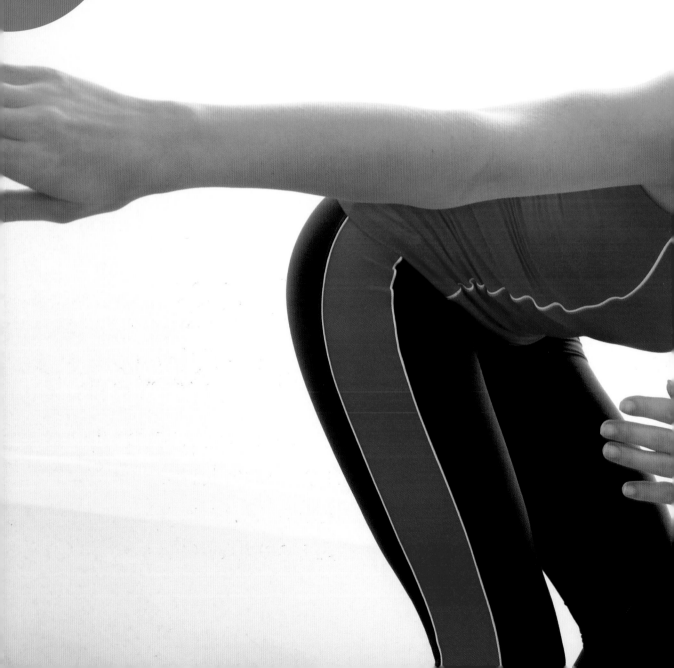

15 minute

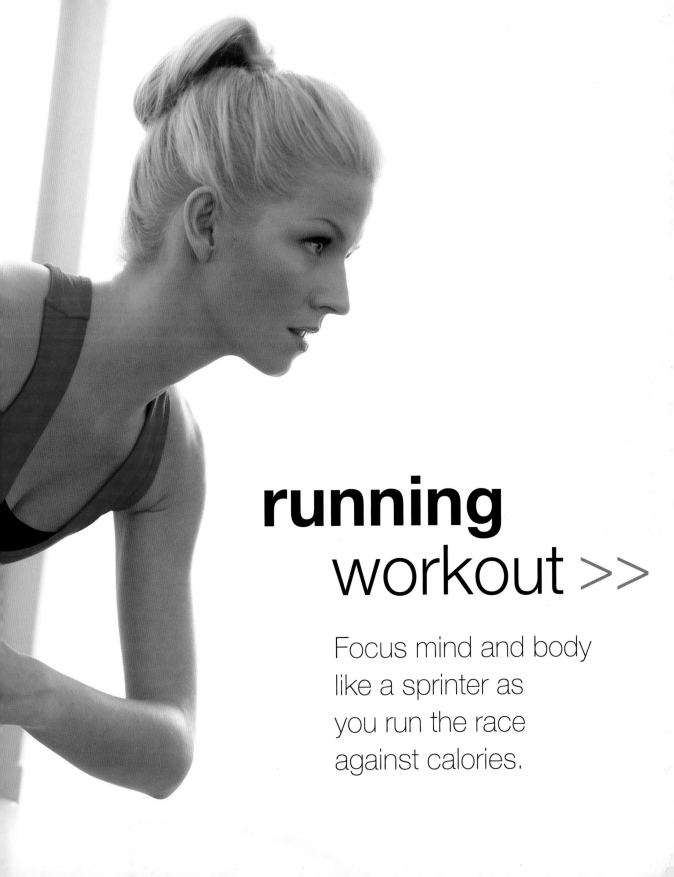

running
workout >>

Focus mind and body
like a sprinter as
you run the race
against calories.

>> **running** workout

Running or jogging outside, especially through a park or on a sandy beach, can't be beaten. Unfortunately, we don't all have those locations on our doorstep, nor an hour or more to spare. So unless you've got a treadmill in your living room, this sequence is the next best thing!

Running is great for your heart and cardiovascular system, and for burning calories, which is why I have included running in this programme. This particular sequence, which incorporates jogging and some sprint-training exercises, is one of the more vigorous workouts in the book. While you are doing it, you'll not only be working out as intensely as you would if you were running outdoors, but you'll also be toning and shaping your muscles.

The downside of running, though, is that your knees and hips undergo a good deal of sustained impact. And for women, there is also the problem of proper bust support. So, before you begin, invest in a good pair of trainers and a sports bra, even if you don't have a big bust.

To keep this running workout as intense as possible and to burn the maximum calories, try to maintain your level of effort throughout. Don't think of the March as less demanding than the Jog, or as an opportunity for a bit of a break. If you really want to burn calories, put ideas like that out of your mind and keep working at a good rate by raising your knees high and really swinging your arms through.

You may think the Step pump is also a good time to catch your breath. Again, if you really want to burn calories, you should intensify your work by exaggerating the contrast between the crouching forward movement and coming back up to standing.

Although the Lunges are performed more slowly than the other steps in the sequence, they are still not an opportunity to take it easy. Lunges are always very taxing, and even more so when you

> ## >> **tips for** your running workout
>
> - **Whenever you land** – for instance, after a hop or a jump – aim for a soft landing with minimum impact. This means keeping your knees soft and rolling through your whole foot, not just landing on your toes.
>
> - **In the Sprint start,** mimic a sprinter at the start of a race. Really power from low to high as you raise your knees towards your chest.
>
> - **In Ski runs,** stay low to the ground, take big steps, and move as far forward and back as you can. In a small space, bend the knees to increase the depth of movement.

have to slow them right down as you do here. To burn those calories, make sure you follow all the tips to get your technique totally perfect and use the concept of "mind to muscle" (see p.106) to help you focus on exactly which parts of your body you are working. Lunges don't just work your thighs. The backs of your legs and your bottom should be working hard, too, so focus your weight into your heels. That will help to remind them to work!

When you're performing this sequence, work your limbs at a good consistent rate and keep your shoulders and neck relaxed as you swing your arms through.

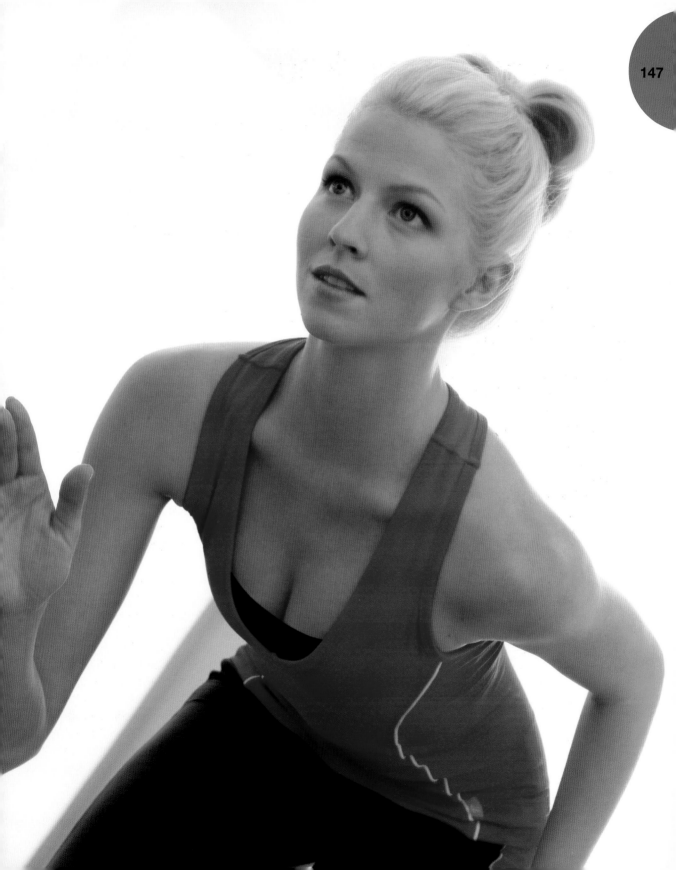

>> deep breaths/half-toe pump

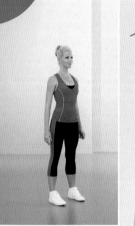

1 Stand tall with feet hip-width apart, knees soft, and arms by your sides. Relax your neck and shoulders, and make sure your tummy is pulled in. Take a deep breath in as you bend the knees and raise your arms above your head. Exhale as you lower them with a smooth circular movement. Make sure your back stays straight. Repeat for a total of 4 reps.

2 Alternate your weight from one foot to the other, rising up onto the ball of your foot. As you alternate feet, curl the opposite arm to your shoulder. Keep your hands in a loose fist and make sure you push your heel right down to the floor as you work your calf muscle. Repeat for a total of 16 reps (1 rep = both sides/directions).

to really lengthen your spine, lift from the hips as you raise the arms upwards

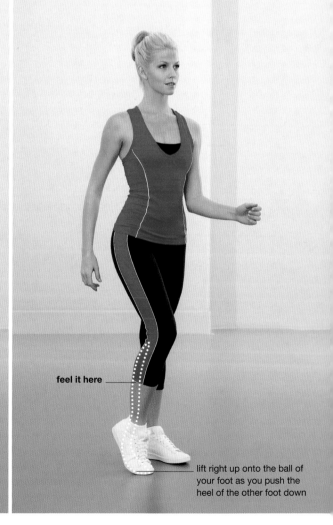

feel it here

lift right up onto the ball of your foot as you push the heel of the other foot down

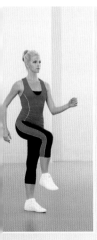

3 Standing on one foot, raise the other knee to waist-height. At the same time, raise the opposite arm. March on the spot, raising opposite knees and arms. Repeat for a total of 8 reps. Then, with your arms by your sides, raise your shoulders towards your ears and roll them in a circular motion, backwards, then forward. Repeat for a total of 4 reps.

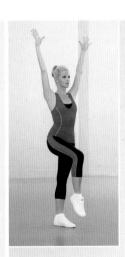

4 Continue marching and, as you do so, stretch your arms sideways to meet above your head, opening and closing your hands at intervals with a "flicking" motion, to warm your fingers and wrists. Continue "flicking" your hands as you lower your arms. Repeat for a total of 4 reps.

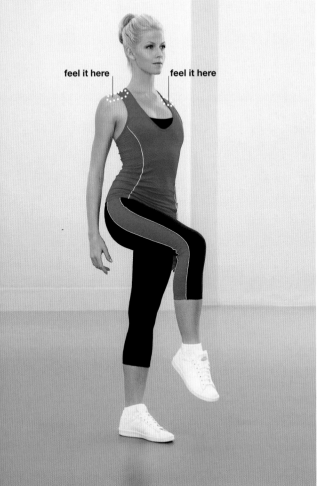

feel it here   feel it here

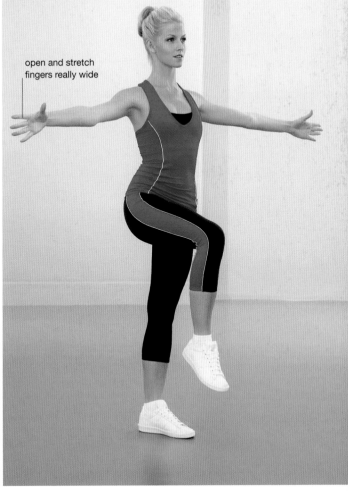

open and stretch fingers really wide

>> **side step/back step**

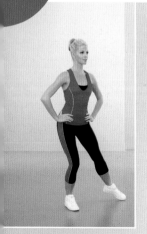

5 With hands on hips, take a step to one side, then bring your feet together. Repeat to the other side. Repeat for a total of 4 reps, then swing your arms in the same direction as you are stepping. Your arms should be relaxed and raised no higher than shoulder-height. Repeat for a total of 8 reps.

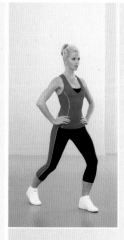

6 With hands on hips, touch one foot on the floor behind you. Return to centre and repeat with the opposite foot. Keep your weight centred as you alternate legs. Repeat for a total of 4 reps, then add an arm push in time with your leg movements by pushing both arms forward and back just below shoulder-height. Repeat for a total of 8 reps.

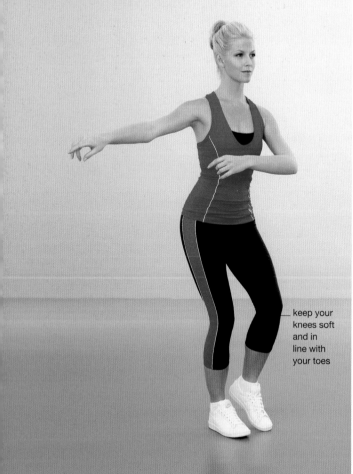

keep your knees soft and in line with your toes

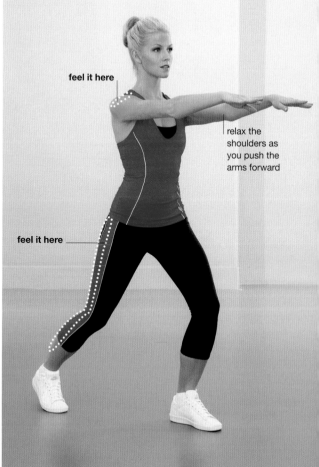

feel it here

relax the shoulders as you push the arms forward

feel it here

>> **dip-kick with twist/roll-up**

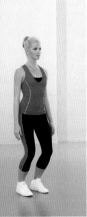

7 With arms by your sides, bend both knees, then come up and kick one foot forward. Repeat for a total of 8 reps, then add a twist by turning your upper body and swinging the opposite arm to the kicking leg. Keep the arms shoulder-height and your hips square. Repeat, alternating sides, for a total of 8 reps.

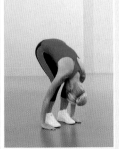

8 Stand tall with feet hip-width apart, arms stretched above your head, shoulders relaxed, and neck and spine in line. Slowly lower your arms and take your chin towards your chest, then round your back and slowly bend down towards the floor. When you are as low as possible, your hands should be relaxed and as near to the floor as is comfortable. Take a deep breath into your lower back. Then, keeping your tummy pulled into your lower back, uncurl slowly, one vertebra at a time, until you have returned to a standing position.

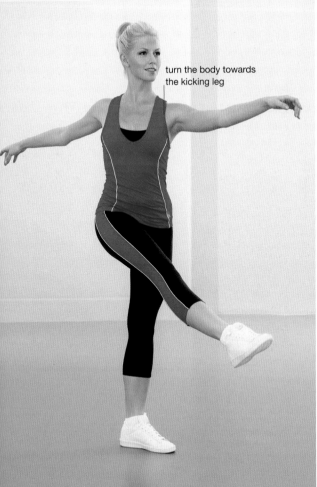

turn the body towards the kicking leg

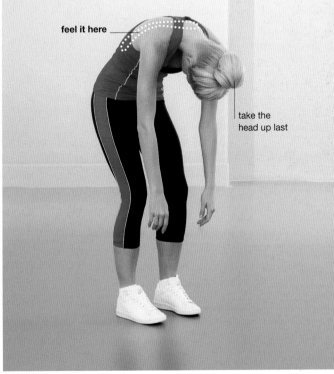

feel it here

take the head up last

>> march/jog

9 Standing on one foot, raise the other knee to waist-height. At the same time, raise the opposite arm. March on the spot, raising opposite knees and arms. Repeat for a total of 16 reps.

10 Curling the opposite arm to the lifted foot, jog on the spot, raising your heels towards your buttocks. Make sure your heels touch the ground every time you land. Repeat for a total of 16 reps.

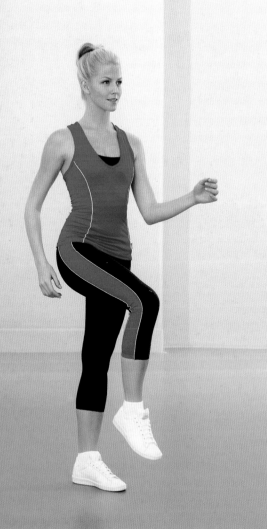

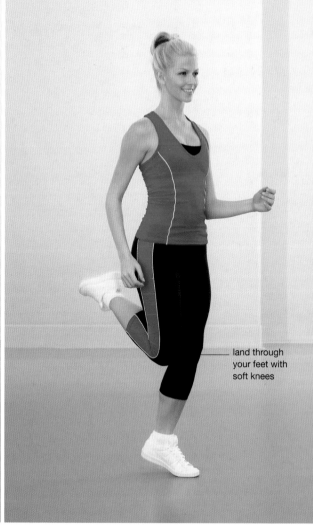

land through your feet with soft knees

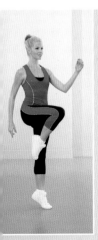

11 Lift one knee towards your chest as you come up onto the toes of the other foot. As you do this, raise the arm opposite to your lifted knee to shoulder-height. The other arm is held slightly behind the body with the elbow soft. Replace the lifted leg to the floor, taking the foot slightly behind and with the knee bent, as you transfer your weight forward. Lift the toe of the opposite leg to flex the foot. Reverse the arms. Repeat for a total of 8 reps, then change sides and repeat for a total of 8 reps.

12 Jump from one leg to the other, lifting your knees high towards your chest. Pump with the opposite arms, so your arm is bent at the elbow and forward on the side of the supporting leg, and slightly bent and backward on the side of the raised knee. Make sure your heels touch the ground every time you land. Repeat for a total of 16 reps. Repeat Step 10.

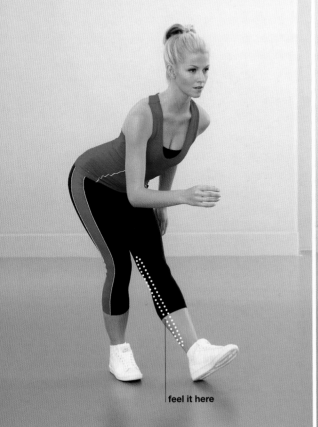

feel it here

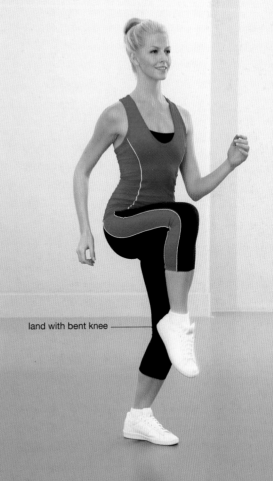

land with bent knee

>> **ski run/half jack**

13 Starting with both feet together, take a diagonal step forward and swing your arms across your body in the same direction. Bring the second foot to the first, then step to the other side and swing your arms the other way. Keep your knees bent and your body low to the ground. Take 4 steps forward, alternating from side to side in a skiing motion, then take 4 steps back in the same way for a total of 8 reps.

14 Starting with both feet together, hands by your sides, and elbows slightly bent, keep one foot planted and step to the side with the other. At the same time, raise both arms above your head. Lower your arms as you bring the foot at the side back to centre, then step to the other side to repeat. Repeat, alternating sides, doing 8 reps.

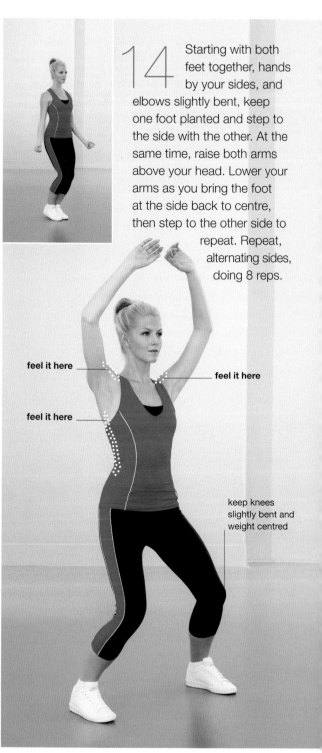

feel it here

feel it here

feel it here

keep knees slightly bent and weight centred

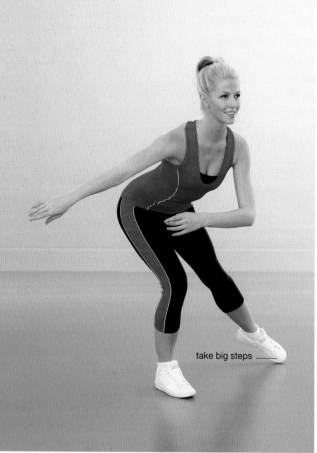

take big steps

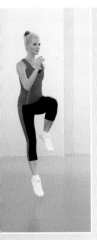

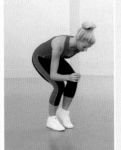

15 Starting with both feet together, hop on one foot as you raise the other knee towards your chest. As you do this, raise the arm opposite to your lifted knee to shoulder-height. The other arm is held slightly behind the body with the elbow soft. Replace the lifted leg to the floor, taking the foot slightly behind and with the knee bent, as you transfer your weight forward. Lift the toe of the opposite leg to flex the foot. Reverse the arms. Repeat for a total of 8 reps, then change sides and repeat for a total of 8 reps. Repeat Step 10.

16 Starting with both feet together, step forward, crouching over one leg with the heel of the other foot raised. Your arm on the side of the raised heel swings slightly behind your body. Your other arm is bent at the elbow. Lower the raised heel as you step back on that foot to an upright position and straighten the other leg. Reverse the arms. Repeat for a total of 8 reps, then change sides and repeat for a total of 8 reps.

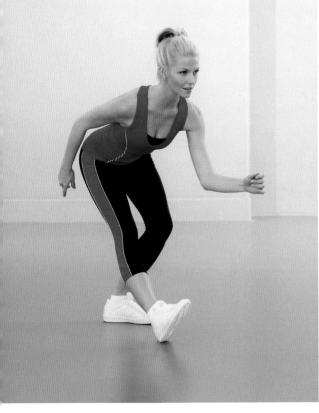

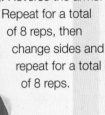

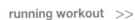

>> lunge/ski run with hop

17 Starting with both feet together, hands on hips, step forward on one foot into a lunge position. Come up, bringing your feet back together, then repeat on the other side. Make sure your hips are square and your knees are in line with your toes. Keep your back straight and your neck and spine in line. Repeat, alternating sides, for a total of 4 reps.

18 Starting with both feet together, take a diagonal step forward, adding a little hop, and swinging your arms across your body in the same direction. Bring the second foot to the first, then step and hop to the other side, swinging your arms the other way. Keep your knees bent and your body low to the ground. Take 4 steps forward, alternating from side to side in a skiing motion, then take 4 steps back in the same way for a total of 8 reps.

Repeat Step 10, then Steps 9–12, then Step 10 again, then Steps 13–15, then Step 10 again, then Steps 16–18, and finally, Step 10 again.

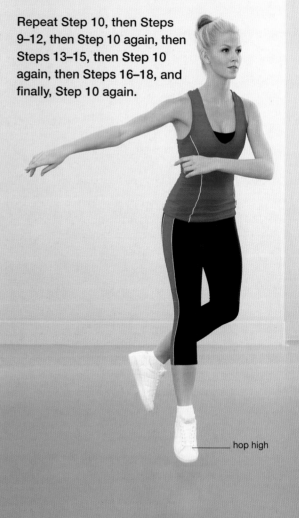

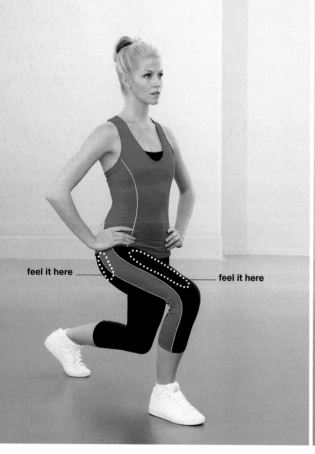

feel it here _____ _____ feel it here

hop high

19 Standing on one foot, raise the other knee to hip-height. At the same time, raise the opposite arm. March on the spot, raising opposite knees and arms. Repeat for a total of 24 reps.

20 Keeping both toes pointing forward, take one leg behind you, and bend the front knee. Clasp your hands in front and raise your arms towards your ears as you lower your head. You should feel a stretch in your upper back, neck, and calf.

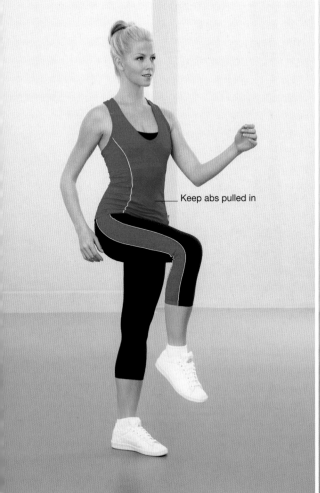

Keep abs pulled in

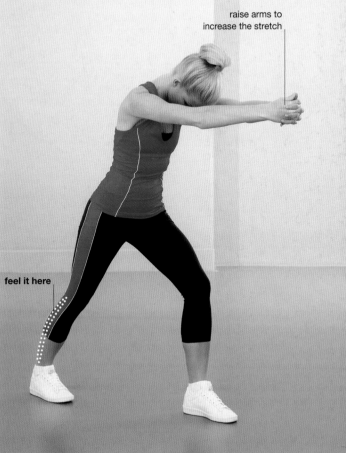

raise arms to increase the stretch

feel it here

>> 3-in-1 stretch 2/quad stretch

21 Take the other leg behind, toes pointing forward, and front knee bent. Clasp your hands behind your back. Open your chest as you raise your arms behind you. You should feel a stretch in your calf, chest, and arms.

22 Stand on one leg and hold the other foot with the hand on the same side. Bring the heel of the raised foot towards the buttock until you feel a stretch in the front of the bent-leg thigh. Change legs. If you cannot keep your balance, hold onto a support.

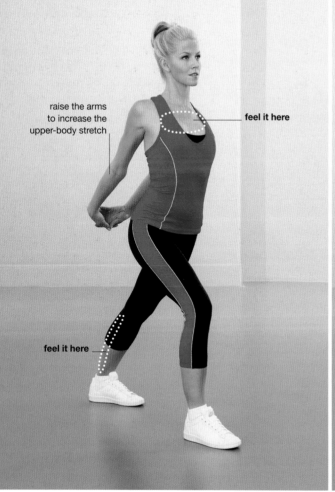

raise the arms to increase the upper-body stretch

feel it here

feel it here

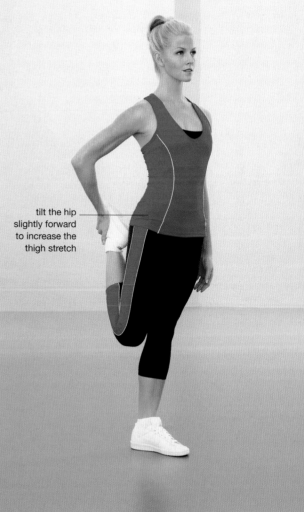

tilt the hip slightly forward to increase the thigh stretch

>> inner-thigh stretch/roll-up

23 Take a step to one side and bend that knee, keeping the knee directly over the toes. Take your hands to the bent-leg thigh and lean forward, stretching the other leg out to the side. Make sure your neck and spine stay in line, and keep your back long and straight. You should feel a stretch in the inner thigh of the outstretched leg. Repeat on the other side.

24 Stand tall with feet hip-width apart, arms stretched above your head, shoulders relaxed, and neck and spine in line. Slowly lower your arms and take your chin towards your chest, then round your back and slowly bend down towards the floor. When you are as low as possible, your hands should be relaxed and as near to the floor as is comfortable. Take a deep breath into your lower back. Then, keeping your tummy pulled into your lower back, uncurl slowly, one vertebra at a time, until you have returned to a standing position.

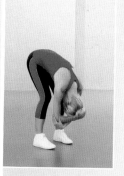

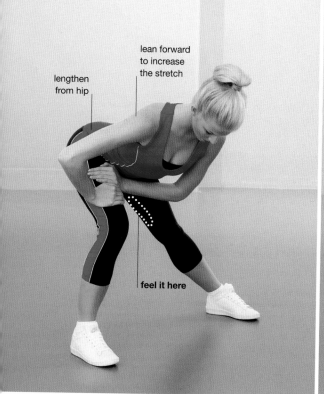

lean forward to increase the stretch

lengthen from hip

feel it here

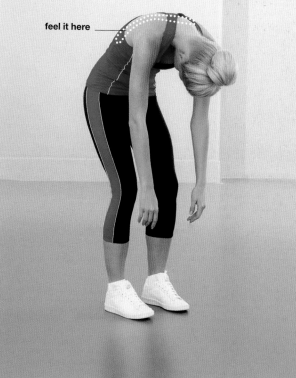

feel it here

running workout at a glance

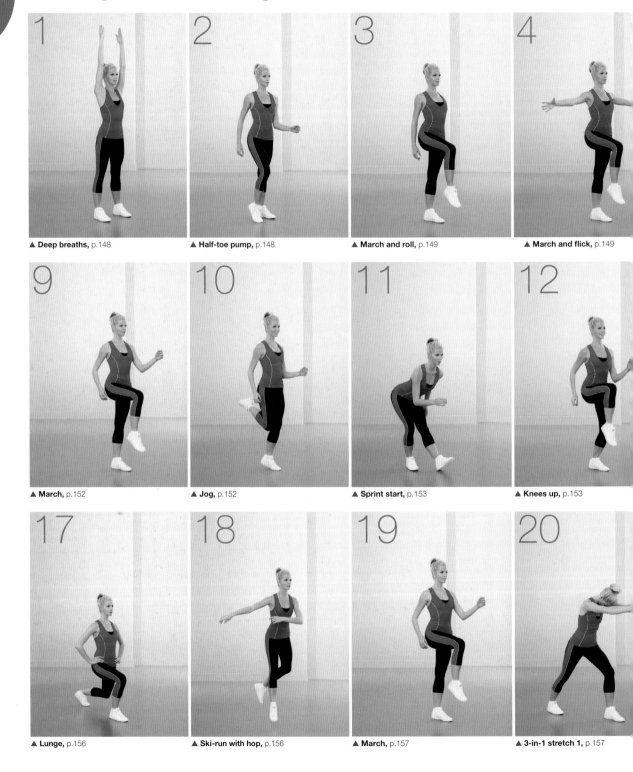

1 ▲ Deep breaths, p.148

2 ▲ Half-toe pump, p.148

3 ▲ March and roll, p.149

4 ▲ March and flick, p.149

9 ▲ March, p.152

10 ▲ Jog, p.152

11 ▲ Sprint start, p.153

12 ▲ Knees up, p.153

17 ▲ Lunge, p.156

18 ▲ Ski-run with hop, p.156

19 ▲ March, p.157

20 ▲ 3-in-1 stretch 1, p.157

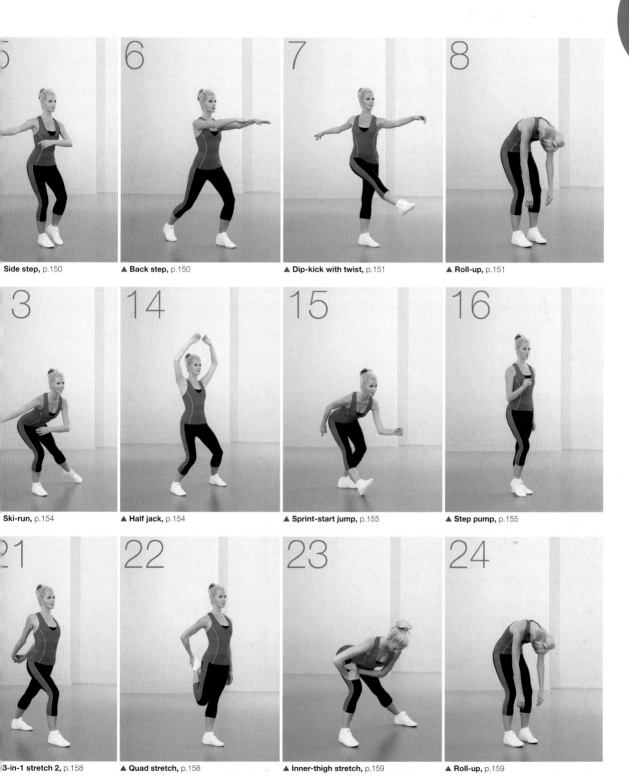

Side step, p.150

▲ Back step, p.150

▲ Dip-kick with twist, p.151

▲ Roll-up, p.151

Ski-run, p.154

▲ Half jack, p.154

▲ Sprint-start jump, p.155

▲ Step pump, p.155

3-in-1 stretch 2, p.158

▲ Quad stretch, p.158

▲ Inner-thigh stretch, p.159

▲ Roll-up, p.159

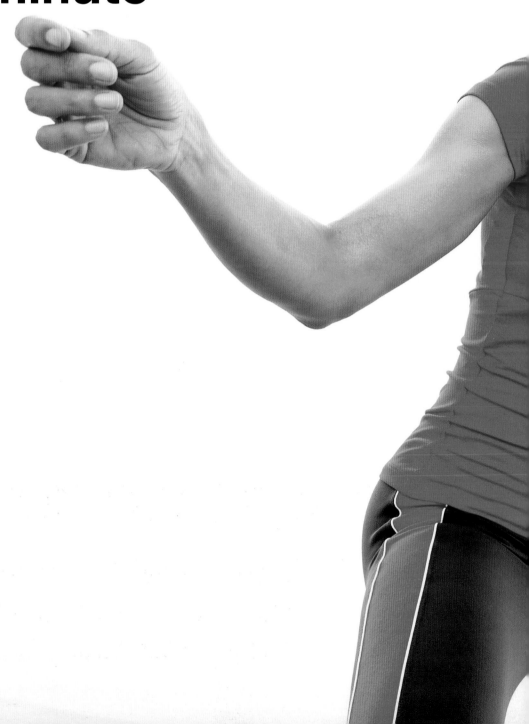

15 minute

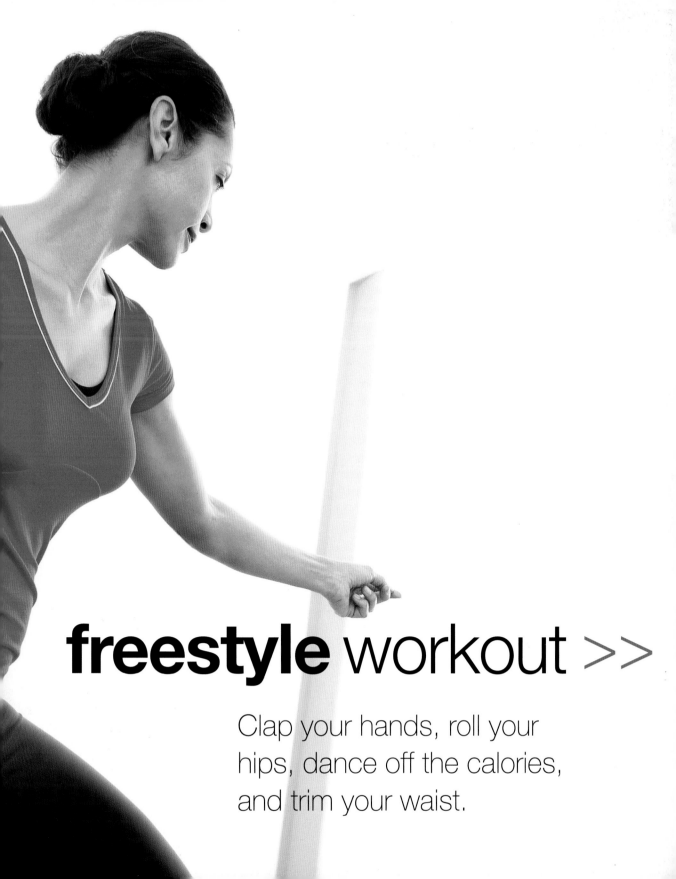

freestyle workout >>

Clap your hands, roll your
hips, dance off the calories,
and trim your waist.

>> **freestyle** workout

I met someone a long time ago who had developed his own workout. Every day he went to his local park, put on his headphones and danced freestyle for an hour to his favourite music. That's what a freestyle workout should be all about, so have fun, and do it like no one is watching.

There are many different styles of freestyle workouts and training – and they are all constantly changing and evolving – so I'm not even going to attempt to list them or compare the benefits of one with another. Suffice it to say that for this particular sequence, I've borrowed moves from two of my favourite freestyle dance styles – disco and reggae. These moves are designed not only for the enjoyment they offer, but also for their good aerobic workout. And you'll certainly appreciate their waist-trimming effect and how they burn the calories.

The best way to intensify this workout and burn extra calories is to let yourself go and really dance your heart out. You'll be surprised how much fun you have and how quickly you feel you've had a worthwhile workout.

Another way is to maintain your posture and form throughout. One thing you will notice about accomplished and professional dancers, regardless of what style of dance they do, is their beautiful posture. Not only does any movement look better when executed with good form and great posture, but it also has a much more beneficial effect on the body in terms of toning and working core muscles.

In fact, a professional dancer's beautiful posture comes from years of core training – strengthening the lower and upper back, and working all the abdominal muscles, including all the deep muscles we can't see. Try to emulate the professionals and you won't fail to burn extra calories. Keep up the effort in your everyday life, and you'll soon notice the difference.

> ## >> **tips for** your freestyle workout
>
> - **As with all training and exercise,** you get back what you put in, so even though this workout may appear to be pretty relaxed, do keep working, stay focused, and really twist your waist.
>
> - **Dancing with company** can boost your fun, so try this dance workout with a friend or partner.
>
> - **Forget you are** even doing any "exercise". Dancing is such an informal way of working your body – especially this relaxed style – so it shouldn't be a chore!

This workout also gives you plenty of opportunity for adding your own special flavour. As soon as you feel you've got the hang of the basic steps, go ahead and add a little hop, or a "shake", or a hand clap. Make it your own. Keep moving. Have a good time. Persuade a friend or partner to get involved, too, and if you've small children, perhaps you can share the moves with them. Watching them doing their own version of the steps can be priceless!

A freestyle dance workout can help you develop and tone your core muscles. It strengthens your upper and lower back, and works wonders for your abdominal muscles, too.

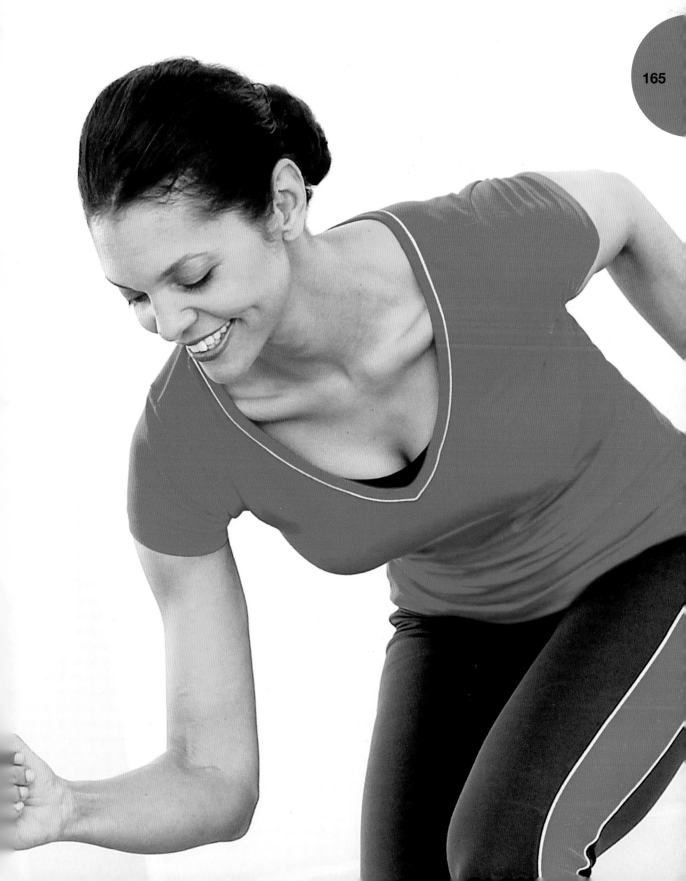

>> deep breaths/half-toe pump

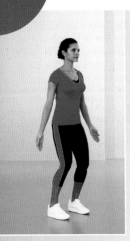

1 Stand tall with feet hip-width apart, knees soft, and arms by your sides. Relax your neck and shoulders, and make sure your tummy is pulled in. Take a deep breath as you bend the knees and raise your arms above your head. Exhale as you lower them with a smooth circular movement. Make sure your back stays straight. Repeat for a total of 4 reps.

to really lengthen your spine, lift from the hips as you raise the arms upwards

2 Alternate your weight from one foot to the other, rising up onto the ball of your foot. As you alternate feet, curl the opposite arm to your shoulder. Keep your hands in a loose fist and make sure you push your heel right down to the floor as you work your calf muscle. Repeat for a total of 16 reps (1 rep = both sides/directions).

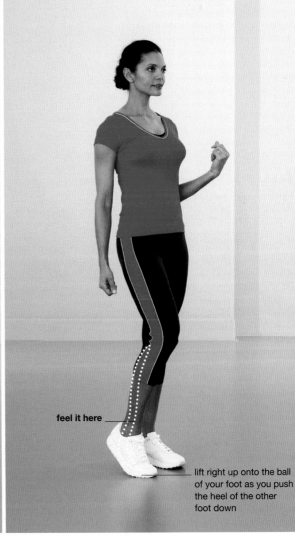

feel it here

lift right up onto the ball of your foot as you push the heel of the other foot down

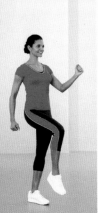

3 Standing on one foot, raise the other knee to waist-height. At the same time, raise the opposite arm. March on the spot, raising opposite knees and arms. Repeat for a total of 8 reps. Then, with your arms by your sides, raise your shoulders towards your ears and roll them in a circular motion, backwards, then forward. Repeat for a total of 4 reps.

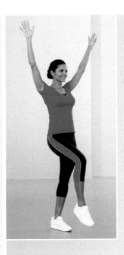

4 Continue marching and, as you do so, stretch your arms sideways to meet above your head, opening and closing your hands at intervals with a "flicking" motion, to warm your fingers and wrists. Continue "flicking" your hands as you lower your arms. Repeat for a total of 4 reps.

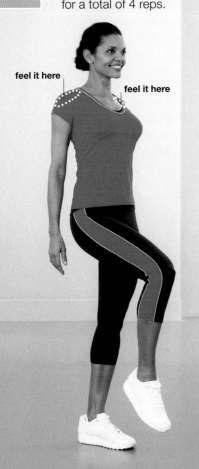

feel it here

feel it here

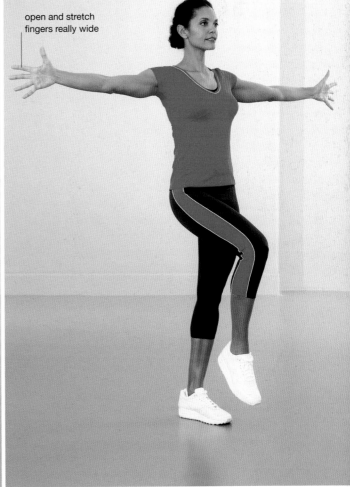

open and stretch fingers really wide

>> **side step/back step**

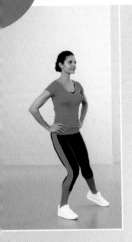

5 With hands on hips, take a step to one side, then bring your feet together. Repeat to the other side. Repeat for a total of 4 reps, then swing your arms in the same direction as you are stepping. Your arms should be relaxed and raised no higher than shoulder-height. Repeat for a total of 8 reps.

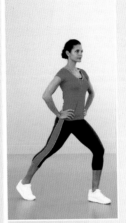

6 With hands on hips, touch one foot on the floor behind you. Return to centre. Repeat with the opposite foot. Keep your weight centred as you alternate legs. Repeat for a total of 4 reps, then add an arm push in time with your leg movements by pushing both arms forward and back just below shoulder-height. Repeat for a total of 8 reps.

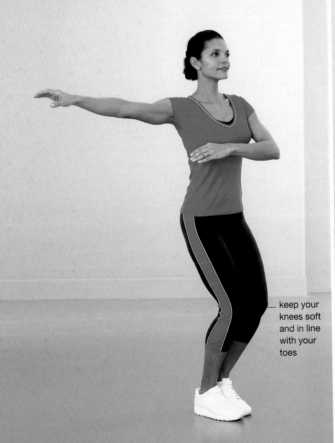

keep your knees soft and in line with your toes

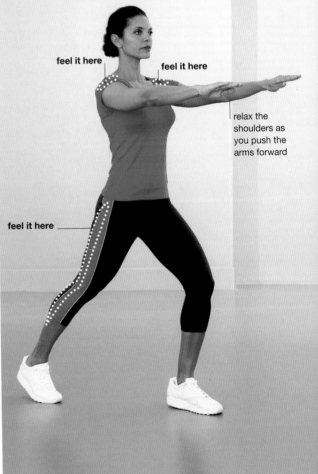

feel it here

feel it here

relax the shoulders as you push the arms forward

feel it here

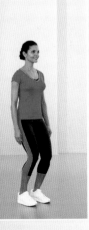

7 With arms by your sides, bend both knees, then come up and kick one foot forward. Repeat for a total of 8 reps, then add a twist by turning your upper body and swinging the opposite arm to the kicking leg. Keep the arms shoulder-height and your hips square. Repeat, alternating sides, for a total of 8 reps.

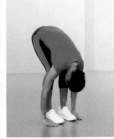

8 Stand tall with feet hip-width apart, arms stretched above your head, shoulders relaxed, and neck and spine in line. Slowly lower your arms and take your chin towards your chest, then round your back and slowly bend down towards the floor. When you are as low as possible, your hands should be relaxed and as near to the floor as is comfortable. Take a deep breath into your lower back. Then, keeping your tummy pulled into your lower back, uncurl slowly, one vertebra at a time, until you have returned to a standing position.

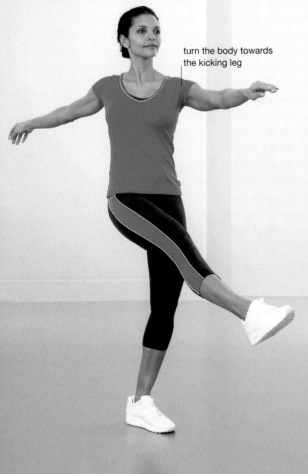

turn the body towards the kicking leg

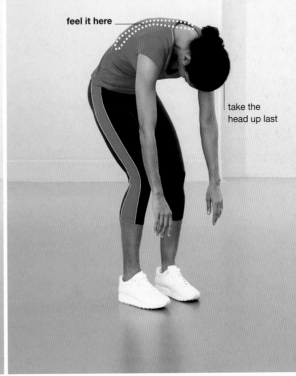

feel it here

take the head up last

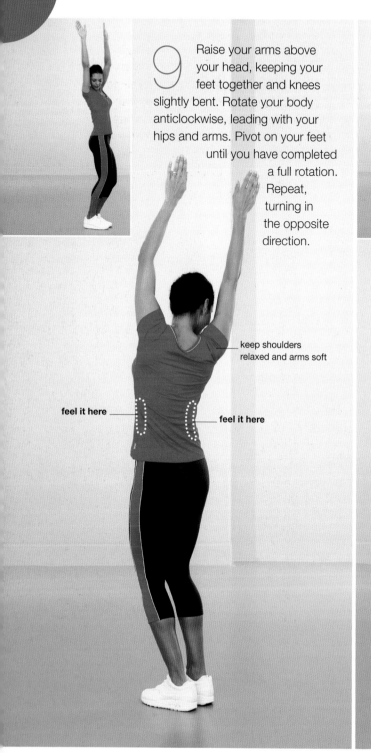

9 Raise your arms above your head, keeping your feet together and knees slightly bent. Rotate your body anticlockwise, leading with your hips and arms. Pivot on your feet until you have completed a full rotation. Repeat, turning in the opposite direction.

keep shoulders relaxed and arms soft

feel it here

feel it here

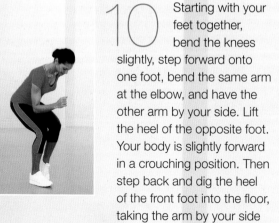

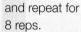

10 Starting with your feet together, bend the knees slightly, step forward onto one foot, bend the same arm at the elbow, and have the other arm by your side. Lift the heel of the opposite foot. Your body is slightly forward in a crouching position. Then step back and dig the heel of the front foot into the floor, taking the arm by your side and bending the other arm at the elbow. Repeat for a total of 8 reps. Change sides and repeat for 8 reps.

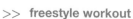

11 With the feet together, take one arm out at shoulder-height, the other in front at chest-height. Twist your hips and swivel, coming up onto the balls of your feet and swinging your arms the other way, then come down and reverse the arms. Continue twisting one way for a total of 4 reps, then change sides and twist the other way for a total of 4 reps. Repeat.

feel it here _____ _____ **feel it here**

12 Starting with the feet together, step forward onto one toe, rotating your hip outwards as you step. The same arm is bent at the elbow behind your body, and the other arm is bent at the elbow in front. Take another step forward on the other foot, rotating the other hip and reversing the arms, then take 2 steps back. Repeat 2 steps forward, 2 steps back for a total of 8 reps. Repeat Step 9.

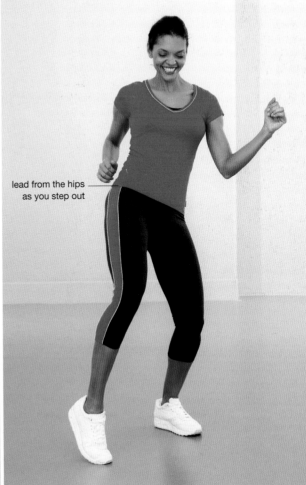

lead from the hips _____
as you step out

>> **step dig and clap/the rock**

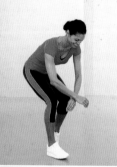

13 Step forward as you crouch over the front leg, both knees bent, and touching the toes of the back foot to the floor. Cross your arms in front of your knees. Step back onto the other leg, digging the front heel into the floor and at the same time raising your hands above your head and clapping. Step backwards and forward for a total of 8 reps, then step forward onto the other foot and repeat.

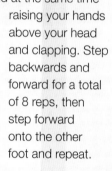

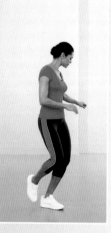

14 Step one leg forward, allowing the other leg to come up onto its toes and bend at the knee. With your elbows bent, let your hands follow the forward step at hip-height. Return that foot to centre and swing your arms the other way. Count "1, 2, 3". Repeat with the other leg. Repeat for a total of 6 reps.

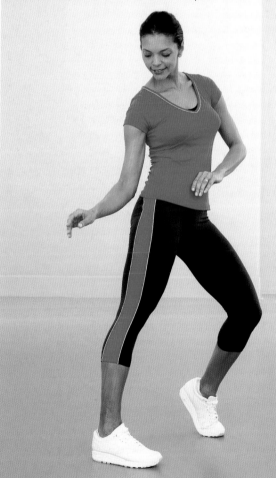

15 Hop onto one leg, raising the opposite knee. Swing the opposite arm forward to shoulder-height and the other arm back. Hop onto the other leg, swinging the arms the other way. Your upper body should follow the motion of the arms as you alternate from side to side. Repeat for a total of 8 reps. Repeat Step 9.

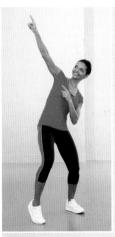

16 Take a step to one side, keeping the other heel raised as you point skywards in the direction of the step. Swing the other arm across your body. Lower your arms to point to the floor as you bring your feet together. Repeat to the same side, then repeat by taking 2 steps to the other side. Repeat, alternating sides, for a total of 8 reps.

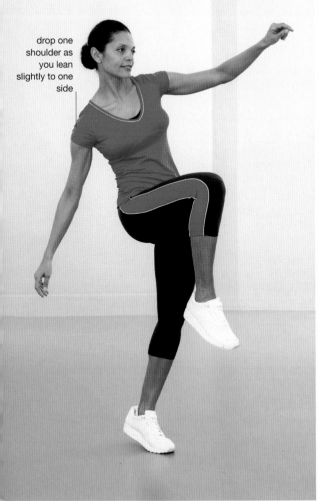

drop one shoulder as you lean slightly to one side

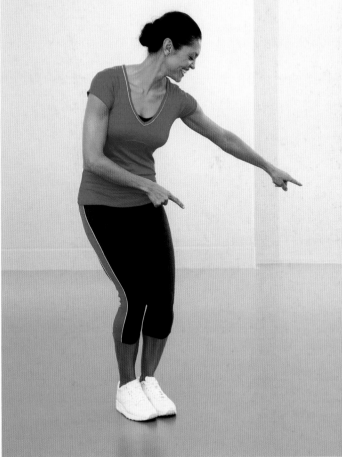

>> heel-dig pump/side-dig swing

17 Starting with feet together, dig one heel forward and raise the toes. Curl the opposite arm to shoulder-height. Repeat, alternating sides, for a total of 16 reps.

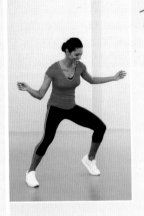

18 Starting with feet together, step to one side, opening both arms out to the sides at chest-height. Return that foot to centre, bending your arms and crossing them in front of your body at waist-height, then repeat to the other side. Repeat, alternating sides, for a total of 8 reps.

Repeat Step 9, then Steps 10-12, then Step 9, then Steps 13–15, then Step 9, then Steps 16–18, then Step 9, then Steps 10-12 again, and finally, Step 9 again.

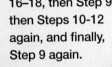

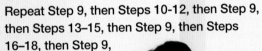

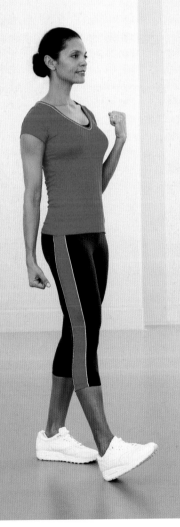

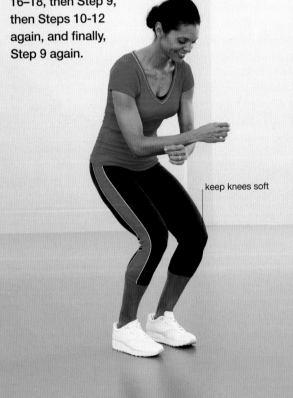

keep knees soft

19 Standing on one foot, raise the other knee to hip-height. At the same time, raise the opposite arm. March on the spot, raising opposite knees and arms. Repeat for a total of 24 reps.

20 Keeping both toes pointing forward, take one leg behind you, and bend the front knee. Clasp your hands in front and raise your arms towards your ears as you lower your head. You should feel a stretch in your upper back, neck, and calf.

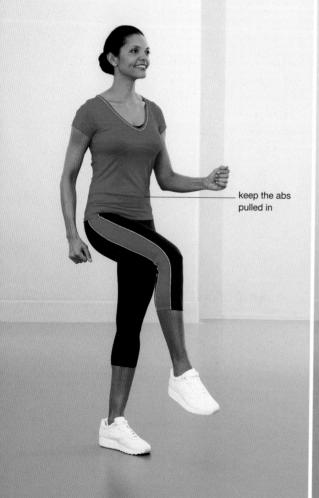

keep the abs pulled in

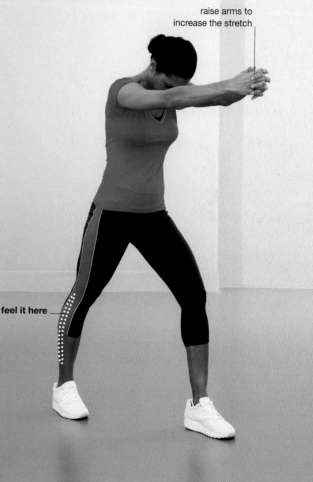

raise arms to increase the stretch

feel it here

21 Take the other leg behind, toes pointing forward, and front knee bent. Clasp your hands behind your back. Open your chest as you raise your arms behind you. You should feel a stretch in your calf, chest, and arms.

22 Stand on one leg and hold the other foot with the hand on the same side. Bring the heel of the raised foot towards the buttock until you feel a stretch in the front of the bent-leg thigh. Change legs. If you cannot keep your balance, hold onto a support.

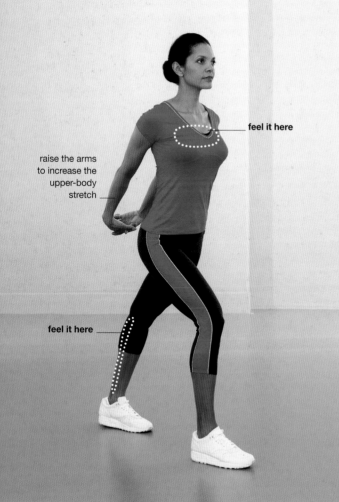

feel it here

raise the arms to increase the upper-body stretch

feel it here

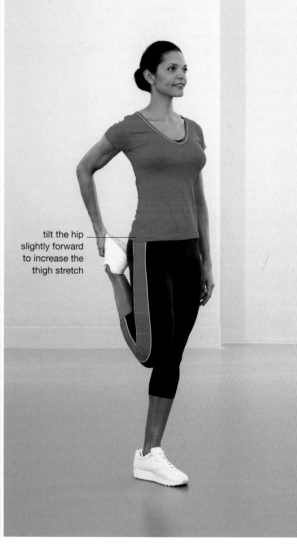

tilt the hip slightly forward to increase the thigh stretch

>> inner-thigh stretch/roll-up

23 Take a step to one side and bend that knee, keeping the knee directly over the toes. Take your hands to the bent-leg thigh and lean forward, stretching the other leg out to the side. Make sure your neck and spine stay in line, and keep your back long and straight. You should feel a stretch in the inner thigh of the outstretched leg. Repeat on the other side.

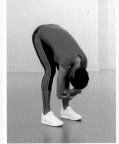

24 Stand tall with feet hip-width apart, arms stretched above your head, shoulders relaxed, and neck and spine in line. Slowly lower your arms and take your chin towards your chest, then round your back and slowly bend down towards the floor. When you are as low as possible, your hands should be relaxed and as near to the floor as is comfortable. Take a deep breath into your lower back. Then, keeping your tummy pulled into your lower back, uncurl slowly, one vertebra at a time, until you have returned to a standing position.

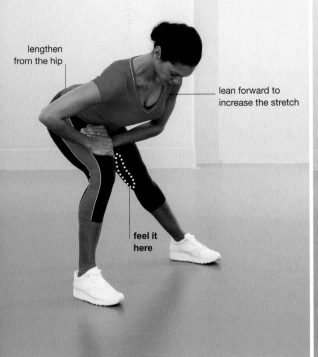

lengthen from the hip

lean forward to increase the stretch

feel it here

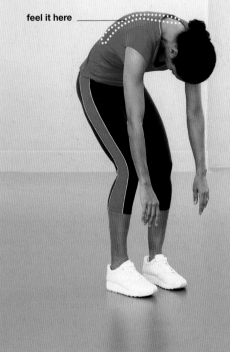

feel it here

freestyle workout at a glance

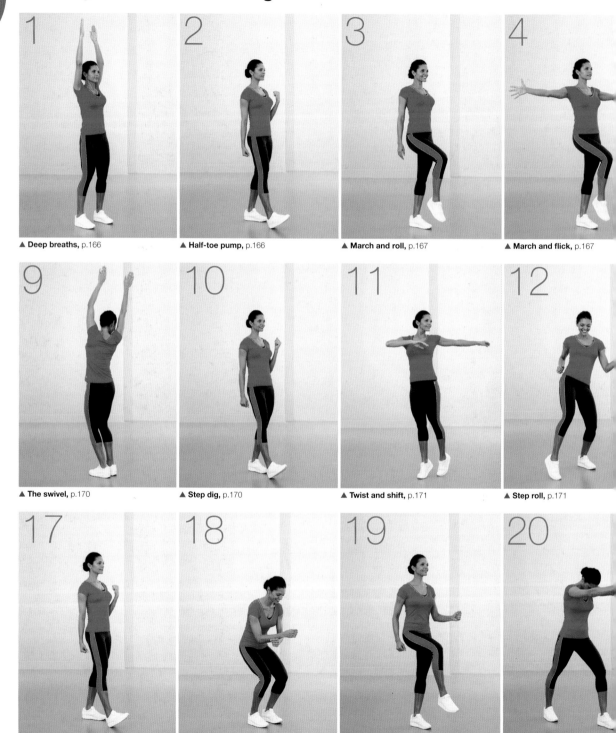

▲ Deep breaths, p.166 | ▲ Half-toe pump, p.166 | ▲ March and roll, p.167 | ▲ March and flick, p.167

▲ The swivel, p.170 | ▲ Step dig, p.170 | ▲ Twist and shift, p.171 | ▲ Step roll, p.171

▲ Heel-dig pump, p.174 | ▲ Side-dig swing, p.174 | ▲ March, p.175 | ▲ 3-in-1 stretch 1, p.175

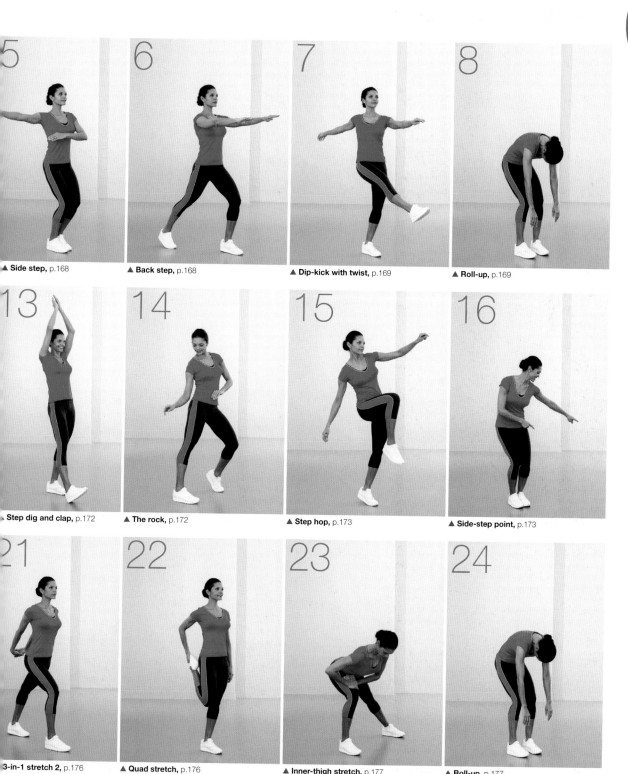

5

▲ Side step, p.168

6

▲ Back step, p.168

7

▲ Dip-kick with twist, p.169

8

▲ Roll-up, p.169

13

Step dig and clap, p.172

14

▲ The rock, p.172

15

▲ Step hop, p.173

16

▲ Side-step point, p.173

21

3-in-1 stretch 2, p.176

22

▲ Quad stretch, p.176

23

▲ Inner-thigh stretch, p.177

24

▲ Roll-up, p.177

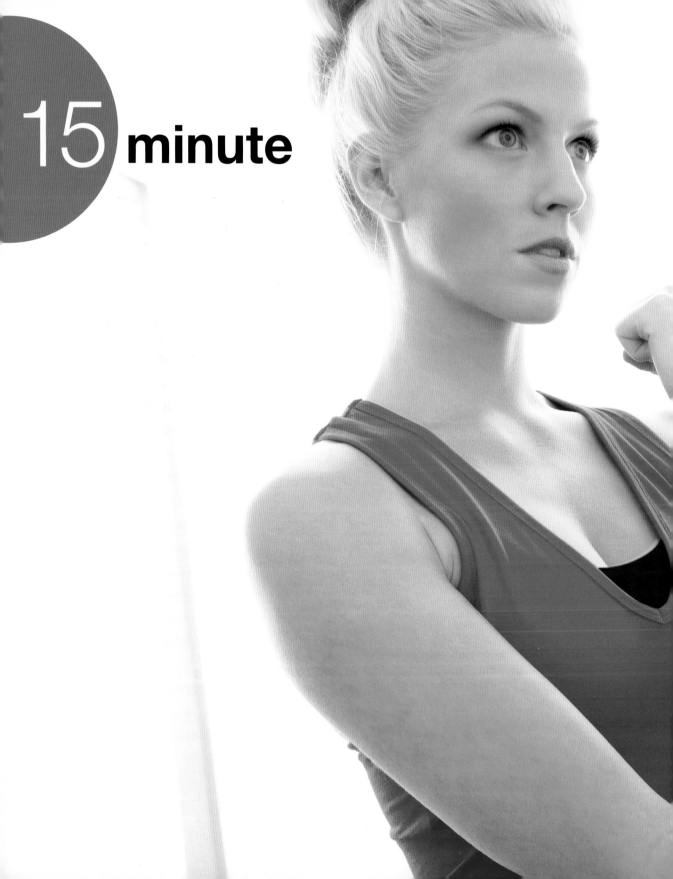

15 minute

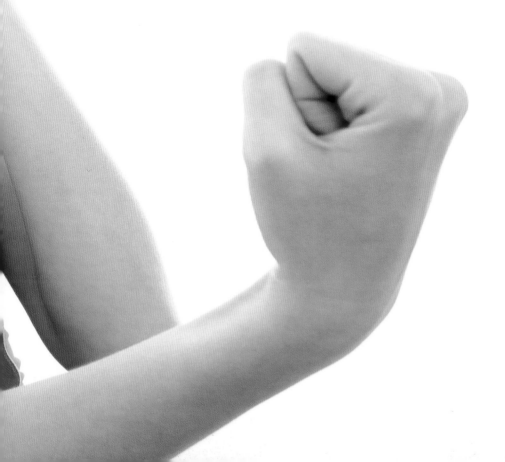

moving on >>

The hardest step is the first, which you've taken. Now it's time to leave your comfort zone and move on to the next level.

>> **boosting** the burn

You're exercising hard and avoiding foods with high sugar and fat content, but somehow you're not losing the weight you want. The problem could be your metabolism. There are aspects of your metabolism that you can influence, so now is the time to work on those.

Metabolism refers to the chemical processes that go on in every cell of our body, enabling us to live and function. Controlled by our hormones and nervous system, metabolism keeps everything working as it should.

None of those chemical processes can take place without energy, and your body gets that, in the form of calories, from the food you eat.

Your Basal Metabolic Rate (BMR; see pp.102–103) is the number of calories your body needs to sustain itself and to function – even when you're sleeping. You also need calories for all your physical activity, whether that's brushing your teeth or training for the Olympics. The bottom line is, if you want to lose weight, you must burn more calories than you take in (eat).

Burning more, burning less

Some of the factors that govern your BMR, such as your sex and age, are out of your control. If you're a man, your body needs more calories a day than if you are a woman. As you get older, your metabolism naturally slows down and uses fewer calories.

If you want to lose weight, you should target those factors you can control. One is your level of physical activity – more exercise burns more calories. The other is your lean-muscle-to-fat ratio. As it turns out, the two are linked. The more you exercise – particularly if you exercise in specific ways (see p.184) – the more lean muscle you'll build, and having a high lean-muscle-to-fat ratio means you'll burn more calories (see p.103). So it's a win-win situation.

>> **boost the burn** unusual facts

- **Too hot? Too cold?** If the ambient temperature is very low or very high, the body has to work harder to maintain its normal body temperature. Naturally enough, this increases your BMR.

- **Stand up for fitness.** Standing uses more energy than sitting, so next time you're standing on the bus, think of it as a mini-workout and enjoy it.

- **Time your eating.** Your metabolism is higher straight after exercise, so if you eat immediately after working out, you will burn more of those calories.

- **Fidgeting pays off.** An American study found that fidgeting produces "non exercise activity thermogenesis". In other words, it burns calories. People in the study with more body fat burned 350 calories less per day than those who were leaner. The leaner people fidgeted more and were generally more active.

- **The male advantage.** Men generally have faster metabolisms than women because they tend to be larger and have less body fat.

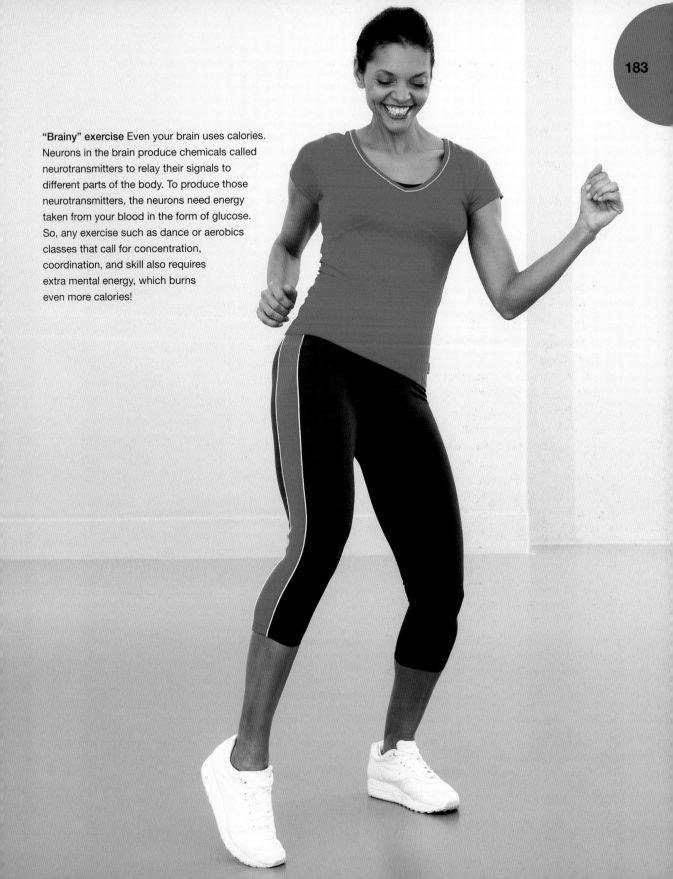

"Brainy" exercise Even your brain uses calories.
Neurons in the brain produce chemicals called
neurotransmitters to relay their signals to
different parts of the body. To produce those
neurotransmitters, the neurons need energy
taken from your blood in the form of glucose.
So, any exercise such as dance or aerobics
classes that call for concentration,
coordination, and skill also requires
extra mental energy, which burns
even more calories!

People often lose muscle as they age, partly because they're less active, so it's good to know that exercise, even when you're older, can reverse the muscle-loss process. When you're older, you can still get results, but you need to work harder for them than when your body was 10 years younger.

Help with staying active

So, if you don't want to gain weight, or if you want to lose it, the key is to increase your level of activity. You may need help to get you started or to keep you moving. If so, there are many professionals you can turn to.

A personal trainer is one. He or she may do some or a combination of the following, according to your needs: a thorough fitness assessment, a specially tailored exercise programme, make regular visits to work with you and check you're staying on track. Of course, a personal trainer is not a low-budget option.

A less expensive choice is to join a gym and work with an instructor there. He or she will show you how to use the various items of fitness equipment safely and will also assess your weight, your percentage of body fat (see p.186), your lung capacity, and your flexibility. You'll be given a tailor-made fitness programme to follow, and every 6 to 8 weeks you can usually have a re-assessment, which will monitor your improvement. Then your fitness programme can be tweaked as required.

Seeing a good osteopath or physiotherapist can also be extremely helpful for getting you on the right track. He or she can identify any problem areas you might have – such as stiff knees or hips – or any that you might develop in the near future, for example if you spend all day hunched over a computer. Such advice is priceless as not only

Resistance training is what you need to help build lean muscle and improve your lean-muscle-to-fat ratio (see p.103). Your muscles have to work against a weight, for example a weighted ball, known as a "medicine ball", as here. Alternatively, you can work against gravity, using use your own body weight in exercises such as squats or press-ups.

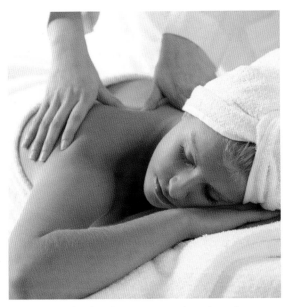

Seeing a professional masseur can be extremely beneficial. A massage helps to get rid of muscle tension, both before and after you work out, and is good for your circulation, too.

can it stop you aggravating existing problems, but it can also help to prevent any condition you are unwittingly heading towards. Your osteopath or physiotherapist can also suggest the type of exercise that would suit you.

Exercise for every age

The World Health Organization defines fitness as "the ability to carry out daily tasks with alertness and efficiency whilst maintaining sufficient energy for leisure pursuits". If you're relatively fit, then this should describe you, and no matter how old you are, you can probably do most types of exercise. Yet some types of exercise may be slightly better for you at certain stages of your life.

Your 20s During our twenties most of us are so busy having fun that we don't realize what an easy ride we're having. We've only recently stopped growing, so our BMR is still relatively high, which means that a little exercise goes a long way.

At this age, you're usually fit enough for any form of exercise, so choose from high-impact cardio (like running and jogging), aerobic exercise,

>> **boost the burn** exercise tips

- **Do resistance training.** Lean muscle mass burns calories (see p.102) and resistance training helps build lean mass. The training works by overloading your muscles – making them perform so they're out of their comfort zone. Use weights or kettlebells at your gym – but be sure you have an induction so you know how to use them correctly. Alternatively, work with resistance bands at home.

- **Vary your exercise.** I've already said that if you don't vary your exercise, you'll reach a "plateau". Then you'll find that you don't feel as satisfied at the end of your workout as you used to. You may also be gaining weight, even if you aren't eating more or exercising less. The reason is that your body has got used to that pattern of exercise, and has become more efficient as it anticipates your exercise programme. So try something else!

- **Add bursts of speed to any aerobic routine.** Known as interval training, this increases your heart rate, which then burns more calories. So, if you're walking, speed up for 20 or 30 seconds, then slow down for a minute or two. Repeat so you add two or three fast-paced intervals and gradually add longer, more intense intervals.

such as cycling or swimming, and resistance training, using your own body weight for doing exercises like squats, sit-ups, or press-ups, or using external resistance, such as a resistance band or free weights.

If you do have any specific issues you need to get to grips with, for example serious weight problems or particularly bad posture, now is the time to do it. Your body is still young and adaptable

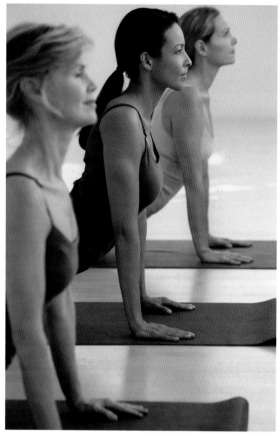

Yoga works whatever your age. The poses stimulate the hormone-secreting endocrine system and help to keep your muscles toned. Yoga's a great stress-buster, too.

and will respond more quickly to change. Make this a time to establish good exercise and eating habits.

Your 30s Between the ages of 28 and 32 is usually when most of us realize that our body "suddenly" isn't the same as it once was. Research has revealed that we naturally lose around 2kg (5lb) of lean body mass and replace it with fat every decade starting from our late 20s. Even if you weigh the same as you did in your 20s, chances are that fat has replaced some of your lean muscle.

Most gyms can take a body-fat reading, or you can buy a machine for home use. If you're female and aged between 20 and 39, a healthy body-fat reading is 21–33 per cent; between 40 and 59, the reading should be 23–34 per cent. If you are carrying extra fat, the longer it's there, the harder

it is to get rid of it. I'm a great believer in aerobic exercise as the best fat stripper, so whatever workout you do, work aerobically in it, which means maintaining a steady pace for a long time.

If you haven't already started resistance training, now's a good time as your bones are already starting to become less dense and this, later in life, can lead to osteoporosis and fractures. Resistance training helps protect you against osteoporosis by slowing down the loss of minerals from your bones while building muscle, too.

Your 40s Whether or not you believe that the 40s are the new 30s, with all the resources we have at our disposal, there's no doubt that you can continue to feel and look great.

You may now need to start toning down your high-impact cardio (running and jogging) to low-impact (brisk walking, rowing, or using a cross trainer) to protect your knees. When walking, keep the aerobic pressure up by pumping your arms as you go or by holding hand weights. You may also want to work your core muscles, to keep – or encourage the return of – your nice flat tummy. Try targeted stomach exercises like crunches or planks, or go to a Pilates class. You should also continue – or start – resistance training exercise.

Also make sure you incorporate stretches in your exercise programme. These not only increase range of movement, but will help tone your muscles. Yoga or Pilates are great for stretching.

Your 50s If you've reached your 50s and never exercised, remember, it's not too late, even though your metabolism will be slowing down (see p.182). If you're a beginner, start by joining a gym and getting your fitness assessed so you're sure to work safely and within your capabilities.

Carry on – or start – resistance training to protect your bones, and do some low-impact cardio such as working on a rowing machine, swimming, or walking, especially uphill.

Finally, don't forget those stretches. If you're lucky, at this stage in your life, you may have more time for yourself, so you can focus on keeping your body in tip-top condition, both now and for many healthy decades to come.

Diet's important, too

As we've seen, calories are units of energy that we get from the food – the carbohydrates, fats, and protein – we eat (see p.102). We take carbs in the form of sugars and complex carbs (bread, grains, beans, vegetables). Fat is usually sourced from oils, butter, meat, and cheese, but there are also high levels of fat in many junk foods, cakes, and biscuits. Protein is supplied by meat, poultry, fish, eggs, cheese, and by some beans and grains, but some of these protein sources also have high levels of fat, so you need to choose carefully.

As a general rule, most people need to take in *less* fat – particularly processed fats found in junk and processed foods – and *less* sugar, caffeine, and alcohol. And it would do most of us good to have *more* complex carbs, fibre (from fruit and vegetables), and water.

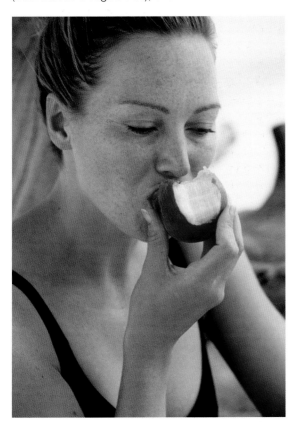

It's now recommended that one-third of your daily food should consist of fruit and vegetables. So there's truth in the old adage "an apple a day keeps the doctor away".

>> **boost the burn** eating tips

- **Eat protein.** Your BMR (see p.102) rises after you eat because it takes energy to eat, digest, and metabolize your food. This is called "thermic effect". The thermic effect varies according to the type of food you eat. Proteins raise your BMR 30 per cent, carbohydrates raise it 6 per cent, while fats only raise it 4 per cent. Clearly, proteins win hands down!

- **Eat hot, spicy foods.** Foods containing chilli, horseradish, and mustard can also have a significant thermic effect, so eating those can raise your BMR.

- **Eat foods that contain iodine.** A diet that's low in iodine reduces your thyroid function, which slows your metabolism. The RDA (recommended daily allowance) is 150mcg. Foods that are richest in iodine are fish and shellfish, but if you happen to be allergic to these, consider taking a supplement. However, too much iodine is also bad for you, so only take a supplement on the advice of a professional practitioner.

- **Eat breakfast.** Your BMR is highest in the morning and tails off gradually through the day, so take advantage of this daily peak. An American study showed that eating a proper meal at the start of the day boosted BMR by 10 per cent and that people who skipped breakfast or lunch had a lower BMR than those who didn't.

- **Don't go on a crash diet.** If you eat too little, your metabolism slows so your body can conserve the energy it's got. Crash dieting can reduce your BMR as much as 15 per cent. Crash dieting also means you lose lean muscle tissue, which in turn reduces your BMR.

>> **broaden** your horizons

Working out in your living room is convenient and is a good place to start, but if your body craves new ways to exercise, you'll probably want to broaden your horizons. The world out there is full of great opportunities for taking your exercise on to the next stage.

Carry on with the good work at home, but now try and make exercise part of your life on a regular basis. Here are some ideas for doing that.

Get out

If you've had fun doing the running workout, you may want to run or jog outdoors. The mistake most people make when they start running is going too fast, and that simply makes them give up. My favourite tip for beginners is "walk a lampost, run a lampost". In other words, run from one lampost to the next, then walk between the following two. When that feels comfortable, and you're ready to push yourself a bit further, try running two lamposts and walking one. If you start to get out of breath, you can always walk two and run one, but be sure to pick up your pace again as soon as you can.

If you're unfit, are carrying a lot of extra weight or have any lower back, knee, or hip problems, it's best to start "low-impact" – marching or walking instead of running or jogging. And if you are older, try walking fast with hand weights or walking uphill rather than running. Both will give you a workout that's as intense as jogging or running.

Get in a pool

Swimming's a great form of exercise as it burns calories without putting any stress on your joints. The water takes the strain, supporting 90 per cent of your body weight. Doing the front crawl is an especially good calorie burner.

But if swimming's not for you, then try aqua aerobics. Essentially, this is aerobic exercise (see p.103) in water. Again, the water supports a large part of your body weight, even though you're exercising in shallow water. A typical class will have you marching, walking and running forward and back, jumping – even doing cross-country ski moves. It's just like doing my running workout (see pp.148–159), but in water.

Go to a gym

Going to a gym gives you the chance to work with different types of equipment. It also helps you to vary the type of exercise you do, which is good for

---

>> **tips for** your next stage

- **When you're outdoors,** run on grass rather than concrete. The strain on your knees will be far less. You'll definitely notice the difference.

- **When you go to the gym,** have an induction by one of the instructors. That way you'll use the equipment safely. You can also ask the instructor to devise a programme that's tailor-made for you.

- **When you join a class,** try to watch one first to be sure it's right for you. Most clubs and lesiure centres allow this.

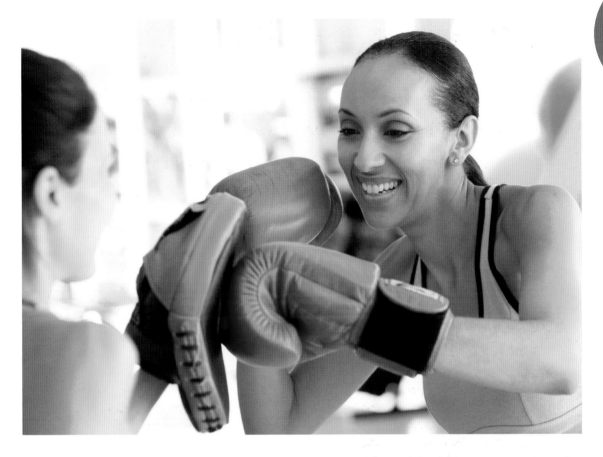

burning calories. If it's more running that you want, you can run on a treadmill, perhaps adjusting the gradient so you can walk "uphill". Other gym equipment that will give you a good cardio workout – one that raises your heart rate, which is good for burning calories – includes stationary bikes, rowing machines, elliptical walkers (also called cross trainers), and stair masters.

Gyms offer a range of strength and resistance training equipment, too. These build muscle and strengthen bones, so helping to guard against osteoporosis. Different machines are designed to work different parts of the body, and you can also work with free weights and kettlebells.

Join a class

If you're ready to take your freestyle dancing, aerobics, or boxing to the next level, joining a class is the way to go. Dance classes come in many shapes and forms, from ballroom, to salsa,

Boxing is becoming more and more popular with women. Boxing with a sparring partner or a punchbag will burn an average 165 calories per 15 minutes.

to hip-hop. They're great fun and a good way of meeting people. Alternatively, go along with a group of friends and burn calories together.

There are also many styles of aerobics classes, but all involve doing routines to music. As you'll have discovered, this is great for helping your motivation and coordination.

And last but by no means least, there are gyms devoted solely to boxing and boxing training. After your 15 minute "taster" you may feel you want to get some boxing gloves on and start punching something. Or you might like to try kickboxing classes – similar to boxing, but using martial arts-style kicks, which give you a good lower-body workout, as well as burning loads of calories.

index

Suzanne Martin

Suzanne is a doctor of physical therapy and a gold-certified Pilates expert. A former dancer, she is a Master trainer certified by the American Council on Exercise. She is published in *Dance Magazine*, *Dance Studio Life*, Dorling Kindersley, and the *Journal of Dance Medicine and Science*, among others. She is also well known within the world of Pilates, dance, and physical therapy. Suzanne is the lead physical therapist for the Smuin Ballet in San Francisco and maintains a private practice, Total Body Development, in Alameda, California. For more information, check her website www.totalbodydevelopment.com

Efua Baker

Efua (pronounced "Ef'wah") started her career as a dancer and fashion model. For more than 15 years she has been a ground-breaking personal trainer or "body sculptor", as she prefers to be called. The focus of her London-based practice has always been to ensure her clients look good and feel great.

Efua has gained a loyal following in the image-driven world of celebrities where her unique and highly effective "body turnaround" techniques are much sought-after.

Efua doesn't just work with famous bodies, she has also developed exercise and motivational programmes for large and diverse groups including new mums, youngsters, and even entire families. It's fair to say she has worked with every type of body there is!

Her workout style draws from many disciplines including dance, body-building, martial arts, yoga, and boxing. Her motto is, "No matter who you are, you are only ever one workout away from looking better and feeling amazing."

Publisher's Acknowledgments

Dorling Kindersley would like to thank Viv Riley at Touch Studios; the models Sam Magee and Tara Lee in Stretching Workout and Carla Collins in Calorie Burn Workout; Rachel Jones, Brigitta Smart, and Victoria Barnes for the hair and makeup; sweatyBetty for the loan of exercise clothing; Peter Kirkham for proofreading, and Hilary Bird for the index.

Picture Credits

The publisher would like to thank the following for their kind permission to reproduce their photographs: Corbis: Comstock p.185; Cathrine Wessel p.103; Getty Images: Image Source p.104; Tetra Images p.186; Photolibrary: Stockbroker p.189.
All other images © Dorling Kindersley
For further information see: www.dkimages.com

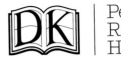

This Edition
Project Editor Kathryn Meeker
Senior Art Editor Glenda Fisher
Editorial Assistant Amy Slack
Jacket Designer Steve Marsden
Photographer Ruth Jenkinson
Creative Technical Support Sonia Charbonnier
Senior Producer, Pre-Production Robert Dunn
Senior Producer Stephanie McConnell
Managing Editor Stephanie Farrow
Managing Art Editor Christine Keilty

First published in Great Britain in 2017 by
Dorling Kindersley Limited
80 Strand, London, WC2R 0RL

Copyright © 2010, 2011, 2017 Dorling Kindersley Limited
Text copyright © 2010, 2011, 2017 Suzanne Martin (pp.10–99)
A Penguin Random House Company
10 9 8 7 6 5 4 3 2 1
001– 298655–Jan/2017

Material in this publication was previously published by DK in *15 Minute Stretching Workout*, 2010; *15 Minute Calorie Burn Workout*, 2010; and *15 Minute Energizing Workout*, 2011.

A CIP catalogue record for this book is available from the British Library.
ISBN: 978-0-2412-8288-5

Printed and bound in China.

All images © Dorling Kindersley Limited
For further information see: www.dkimages.com

A WORLD OF IDEAS:
SEE ALL THERE IS TO KNOW

www.dk.com